# Convection Oven Cookbook

*Convection Oven Cookbook: Delicious and Easy Recipes for Crispy and Quick Meals in Less Time and Easy Cooking Techniques for Any Convection Oven*

## Stephanie Robbins

© Copyright 2020 by (Stephanie Robbins)- All rights reserved.

This document is geared towards providing exact and reliable information regarding the topic and issue covered. The publication is sold with the idea that the publisher is not required to render accounting, officially permitted or otherwise qualified services. If advice is necessary, legal or professional, a practiced individual in the profession should be ordered.

- From a Declaration of Principles which was accepted and approved equally by a Committee of the American Bar Association and a Committee of Publishers and Associations. In no way is it legal to reproduce, duplicate, or transmit any part of this document in either electronic means or printed format. The recording of this publication is strictly prohibited. Any storage of this document is not allowed unless with written permission from the publisher. All rights reserved.

The information provided herein is stated to be truthful and consistent. In terms of inattention or otherwise, any liability, by any usage or abuse of any policies, processes, or Steps of preparation contained within is the recipient reader's solitary and utter responsibility. Under no circumstances will any legal responsibility or blame be held against the publisher for reparation, damages, or monetary loss due to the information herein, either directly or indirectly. Respective authors own all copyrights not held by the publisher. The information herein is offered for informational purposes solely and is universal as so. The presentation of the information is without a contract or any guarantee assurance. The trademarks used are without any consent. The publication of the trademark is without permission or backing by the trademark owner. All trademarks and brands within this book are for clarifying purposes only and are owned by the owners themselves, not affiliated with this document.

# Table of Contents

Introduction ........................................................................................................................ 7

**Chapter 1: Basics of convection Oven** ........................................................................ 9

    *1.1 What is a convection oven?* ...................................................................................... 9

    *1.2 Convection versus conventional oven* ................................................................... 10

    *1.3 Convection is ideal for baking* ................................................................................ 11

    *1.4 Convection oven for roasting* .................................................................................. 12

    *1.5 Things to remember when cooking in a convection oven* ................................... 13

    *1.6 Converting the Convection Oven Recipes* ............................................................ 13

**Chapter 2: Different types of convection ovens and their usage** ........................ 14

    *2.1 Culinary Ovens with Convection* ........................................................................... 14

    *2.2 Other varieties of convection oven* ........................................................................ 15

    *2.3 Convection ovens for commercial applications* ................................................... 16

    *2.4. Convection ovens for customers* ........................................................................... 16

**Chapter 3: When and when not to use convection oven?** ..................................... 17

    *3.1 Why should the convection setting be used?* ....................................................... 17

    *3.2 When to use the convection setting?* ..................................................................... 17

    *3.3 The Convection Configuration when not to be used* .......................................... 18

    *3.4. How to utilize the Environment of Convection* ................................................. 18

    *3.5 Drawbacks of convection oven* .............................................................................. 19

**Chapter 4: Convection Oven Chicken recipes** ........................................................ 21

    *4.1 Chicken Broast* .......................................................................................................... 21

    *4.2 Convection oven chicken wings* ............................................................................ 22

    *4.3 Chicken and Potatoes Oven Roasted* .................................................................... 23

    *4.4 Baked simple Chicken Breasts* ............................................................................... 25

    *4.5 Chicken veggie dish* ................................................................................................. 26

    *4.6 Lemon Garlic Roasted Chicken and Potato Wedges* .......................................... 27

    *4.7 Oven-Fried Extra Crispy Chicken Thighs* ............................................................ 28

    *4.8 Rotisserie styled chicken* ......................................................................................... 28

    *4.9 Crispy convection Oven Baked Chicken Wings* .................................................. 30

    *4.10 convection Baked Chicken Drumsticks* .............................................................. 31

    *4.11 Baked Chicken Thighs Perfect Crispy* ................................................................. 32

*4.12 Lemons and Garlic Roast Chicken* ........................................................................................... 33

*4.13 Crispy Oven Chicken Tenders* ................................................................................................. 34

*4.14 Roasted Chicken with Lemon Garlic flavored Potato Wedges* ................................................ 35

*4.15 Pepper chicken with potato wedges* ........................................................................................ 36

*4.16 Golden Roast Hens with delicious vegetable hash* .................................................................. 36

## Chapter 5: Beef and lamb .............................................................................................................. 39

*5.1. Prime Rib* .................................................................................................................................. 39

*5.2. Honey Pork Chops Grilled* ....................................................................................................... 40

*5.3. Sicilian-style Strata* .................................................................................................................. 41

*5.4. South-west Cheese Puff Pot Beef Pie* ...................................................................................... 42

*5.5. Meatloaf* .................................................................................................................................... 44

*5.6 Easy Calzone* ............................................................................................................................ 46

*5.7 Meatballs* ................................................................................................................................... 46

*5.8 Prosciutto Roast Pork Tenderloin* ............................................................................................. 47

*5.9 Perfect Beef Jerky* ..................................................................................................................... 49

*5.10. Roast Leg of Lamb with Herbs* ............................................................................................... 50

*5.11. Lamb Shanks with Olives and Capers* ................................................................................... 51

*5.12. Roast Beef* ............................................................................................................................... 52

## Chapter 6: Desserts ....................................................................................................................... 54

*6.1. Convection Spooky Cake* ......................................................................................................... 54

*6.2. Brie Filo-wrapped* .................................................................................................................... 56

*6.3. Choco Nut Brownies* ................................................................................................................ 57

*6.4 Chocolate chip cookies* ............................................................................................................. 58

*6.5 Christmas Magic Bars* .............................................................................................................. 59

*6.6 Creme Brule* .............................................................................................................................. 60

*6.7 Olive Oil Granola with cherries and pecans* ........................................................................... 60

*6.8. Gingersnap Baked Apples* ........................................................................................................ 61

*6.9 Pear and Ginger Cake* .............................................................................................................. 62

*6.10. Louisiana Pecan Balls* ............................................................................................................ 64

*6.11 Fresh Peach Pie Rock Creek Lake* .......................................................................................... 65

*6.12 Sweet and Hot Spiced Pecans* ................................................................................................. 66

*6.13 Leek and Dubliner scones* ....................................................................................................... 67

*6.14 Roasted Potato Rosemary Idaho with Apple Salad* ................................................................ 68

*6.15 Oat Bars Very Berry* ................................................................................................................ 69

 6.16 Blossom Panna Cotta Yogurt-Orange ............................................................................... 71

 6.17 Quinoa Sticky Toffee Pudding ............................................................................................ 74

 6.18 Sour Cream Cardamom Cake ............................................................................................ 76

## Chapter 7: Turkey .............................................................................................................. 78

 7.1 Turkey Picnic Loaf Jerk-spiced ............................................................................................ 78

 7.2. Classic Roast Turkey ........................................................................................................... 80

 7.3. Thanksgiving Mayonnaise Roasted Turkey ..................................................................... 81

 7.4. Rosemary and thyme flavored turkey .............................................................................. 82

 7.5. Spatchcocked Turkey served with Herb Butter and Flavored Gravy ........................... 82

## Chapter 8: Fish ................................................................................................................... 85

 8.1 Fish Tacos .............................................................................................................................. 85

 8.2. Grilled Garlic Salmon .......................................................................................................... 86

 8.3 Fish Parsley Pesto .................................................................................................................. 87

 8.4 Homemade Fish Sticks ......................................................................................................... 88

 8.5 Baked Parmesan Swai .......................................................................................................... 88

 8.6 Garlic Roasted Mahi Mahi ................................................................................................... 89

 8.7 Geraine's Mahi Mahi Ginger Soy ........................................................................................ 90

## Chapter 9: Pizza .................................................................................................................. 92

 9.1 Cheese Pizza Recipe ............................................................................................................. 92

 9.2 Vegetable pizza ..................................................................................................................... 93

 9.3 Chicken cheese pizza ............................................................................................................ 96

## Chapter 10: Snacks ............................................................................................................. 99

 10.1. Oven fries ........................................................................................................................... 99

 10.2. Roasted potatoes ............................................................................................................... 100

 10.3. Simple Bacon ..................................................................................................................... 101

 10.4. Popovers ............................................................................................................................. 102

 10.5. Convection Oven Granola ................................................................................................ 103

 10.6. Roasted vegetables ............................................................................................................ 105

 10.7. Christmas Magic Bars ....................................................................................................... 106

 10.8 Grilled veg sandwiches in the oven ................................................................................. 107

 10.9 Oven-Roasted Spicy Fries ................................................................................................. 108

 10.10 Garlic roasted potatoes ................................................................................................... 109

 10.11 Roasted butternut squash ............................................................................................... 110

10.12 Oven Roasted Cauliflower Recipe .................................................................................. 111

10.13 Brussel sprout parmesan ................................................................................................ 112

10.14 Spaghetti squash ............................................................................................................ 113

10.15 Asian-Inspired Shepherd's Pie ...................................................................................... 113

## Chapter 11: Bread recipe ........................................................................................................ 115

11.1 Homemade Bread ............................................................................................................ 115

11.2 Cinnamon flavored banana bread ................................................................................... 116

11.3 Brown bread ..................................................................................................................... 117

11.4 Simple banana bread ....................................................................................................... 119

## Chapter 12: Miscellaneous ..................................................................................................... 121

12.1 Oven-roasted root veggies ............................................................................................... 121

12.2 Stacked Enchilada Pie ..................................................................................................... 122

12.3 Golden rice crisps ............................................................................................................ 124

12.4 Apple and Endive Salad with Honey Vinaigrette .......................................................... 125

12.5 Endive casserole .............................................................................................................. 125

## Conclusion ............................................................................................................................... 128

# Introduction

A traditional oven usually cooks by covering the food in hot and dry air. The hot air heats external surface of the food; the heat is then directed from outside towards the food's inside until it is cooked completely. In other words, the food's outer areas get heated, while the inner portion of the food is heated by the already-heated outer area adjacent to it. It means that the food cooks itself. However, outer parts are more exposed to higher temperatures. That is why roast is brown and also crusted from the outside, but it is still medium-rare from the center. The oven's air might be almost 400 F, but the roast's center is 135 F.

The fan generates additional energy in the convection oven. It takes and blows the hot air through it, raising the intensity with which hot air hits the roasting surface. For example, when you stand inside a hot bath or swirled some water around yourself, the water feels cooler when it falls against the legs. However, the feeling of extra heat disappears when you avoid swirling it. That is the convection effect, though with the fan.

A question which may come to your mind is how much excess energy is required in convection oven? The answer is it depends on the strength of the fan. Convection ovens generate about 25 to 30 % more electricity. It is necessary to quantify this extra energy in terms of temperature or cooking period. Another question that you may be thinking is does the convection oven work hotter than a traditional oven. Or is it easier to cook? The response to that is both.

Certain convection ovens provide different baking and roasting configurations. The two points to note are: its extra energy generated by a convection oven falls in the context of heated, whooshing air, and since this whooshing air can come into contact with a surface of your food, it will be the surface of the food that will bake faster inside a convection oven. The inside of the food would not experience this air, and although radiant heat of the oven will similarly cook. What does it imply? In brief, for roasting broad pieces of beef where you like them to be nicely browned from the outside yet medium rare from the inside, convection ovens are fantastic. In general, this means beef roasts, especially prime ribs, lamb legs, and, to a lesser °, pork (that should be cooked medium instead of medium). This book will cover everything you need to know about convection oven and all the related concerns. It will also provide you with some delicious recipes of chicken, meat, snacks, salads, fish etc. So, lets start learning convection oven basics, its working and then start making some delicious easy to make recipes.

# Chapter 1: Basics of convection Oven

If your oven has a convection feature, lift your hand. Now, if you have no idea when or how to use it, hold your hands up because this book is the right place for you. There must be many questions lingering in your mind regarding convection oven usage and what exactly is its function. How exactly convection oven works? How it is different from conventional oven? With the convection setting, can we bake? When and when not to use convection oven for cooking?

Questions are too many! Let's work out what convection is, learn about when it can be used, and, more importantly, when it should not be used.

## 1.1 What is a convection oven?

The convection oven is nowadays very famous for cooking purposes. Simply stated, there is a fan and exhaust mechanism in the convection oven. The fan and the exhaust aid in blowing the hot air around and over the food, then exhaust it back outside. Consequently, the food is surrounded by the hot air, such that it heats uniformly at the surface more proficiently.

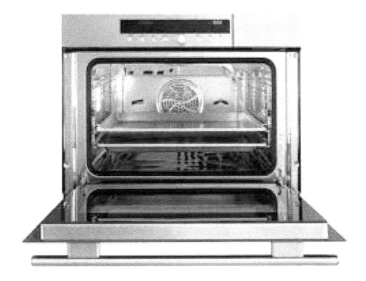

To better clarify this, ponder on the example of wind chill: On a blustery winter day, as cold air blows toward you, you get warmer quicker than you would on a windless day with the same weather. The same relates to convection system. The fan generates additional energy in the convection oven. It takes and blows the hot air through the food, practically raising the intensity with which the hot air hits the roasting surface.

Another example is a hot bath. The water feels cooler when it falls against your legs, when you stand in a hot bath and swirl the water around yourself. However, the feeling of extra heat goes away when you avoid swirling it, this is called the convection effect. With the fan it is the same effect as the convection oven makes.

One of the specifications of convection oven includes the strength of the fan. In convection ovens 25 to 30 percent more energy is generated. It is necessary to quantify this extra energy in terms of temperature or cooking period. The heat in a convection oven is constant regardless of the presence of fan and extra energy.

## 1.2 Convection versus conventional oven

When you are moving into a completely new home or if you choose to renovate your existing kitchen, there are two options when selecting an oven. It is either a traditional oven or the convection oven. What is the distinction between the two of them?

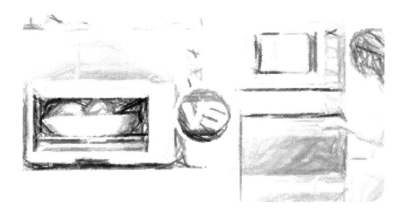

By enveloping food in thick, dry air, an ordinary oven cooks the food. This hot air covers the surface of the food, so this heat is carried from the outside of the food into the food's interior until it is cooked well all the way inside. To describe it in another way, the exterior areas of the food are heated by the oven, while the inner parts are heated by the outer regions that are parallel to the parts of the food which are already heated. In this way, the food is heating itself. But the outside sections are subjected to higher temperatures. Consequently, on the top, roast will be brown and crusted, but it is always medium-rare in the middle. The air maybe 400 F in the oven, but the middle of the roast is 135 F.

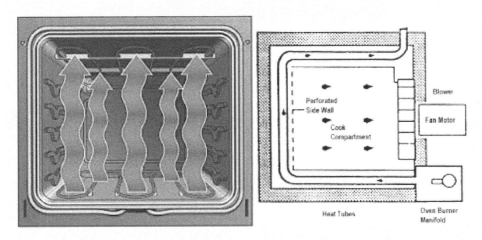

Conventional vs convection oven heating

## 1.3 Convection is ideal for baking

The heat is spread uniformly all over the food in a convection oven. Professional cooks prefer convection oven for baking because it cooks food uniformly and 25 percent quicker than a traditional oven. A convection oven often doesn't need to be preheated compared to traditional oven and hence considered as a good option for baking.

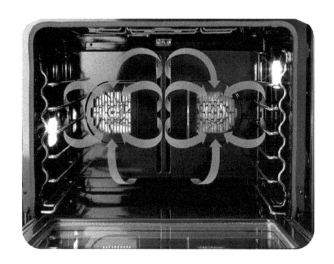

## 1.4 Convection oven for roasting

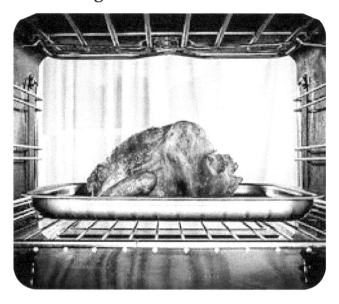

When roasting meat, it is necessary to make some adjustments with the recipes. The convection effect will dry out the meat surface and additional heat may damage the protein fibers. Higher average temperature will cause roasts to shrink more compared to ordinary ovens.

On the other side, turkey and chicken are cooked well from both outside and inside. But you have a choice of decreasing the temperature or reducing the cooking period with a convection oven. Just be sure that chicken's leg deepest section is thoroughly roasted, and the wind is not blowing there. You are best off reducing the temperature in this case and keeping the cooking period the same.

## 1.5 Things to remember when cooking in a convection oven

Two things that should be noted are:

- The convection oven generates the extra energy in the form of thick, whooshing air.
- The surfaces of the food that comes in touch with the whooshing air will be cooked more rapidly in convection oven.

This hot air will not penetrate the cooking interior since the oven's heat generated will concurrently cook food in a normal manner. In brief, convection ovens are fantastic for roasting broad meat pieces when you like them to be perfectly browned from the outside but medium rare from the inside. This refers to beef roasts, especially prime ribs, as well as lamb legs, and, to a lesser degree, pork.

## 1.6 Converting the Convection Oven Recipes

Today, for the traditional ovens, virtually for any recipe temperatures and the cooking times are specified. But in the convection oven cooking, it is suggested that you have to convert the recipe. This requires decreasing the temperature or shortening the cooking period is required for every recipe. Setting the oven 25 to 50 ° less than the recipe suggests is the easiest process. In the case of 400 F, you have to decrease to 375 to 350 F.

There are certain convection ovens which adjusts the heat change by themselves. For example, if you adjusted the convection oven at 350, it will simply set itself to 325. You should keep the temperature same and just shorten the cooking period by 25 percent (assuming your oven does not self-correct). But when baking cookies and pies, reduce the temperature to 25 °. Keep the temperature decrease to 50 ° when roasting the meat. Convection ovens are provided with a manual which can guide much about these heat adjustments and configurations.

# Chapter 2: Different types of convection ovens and their usage

The word "convection" is generally used to indicate "fan-assisted". However, this may not be the most appropriate way to discern fan-based ovens over traditional ovens. All forms of oven work utilizing convection (heat transfer due to hot air bulk movement). The traditional ovens circulate the hot air, and the fan-assisted ovens distribute the hot air using artificial convection. The word "convection" is scientifically applicable to both the conventional ovens and the fan-assisted ovens. However, difference between the traditional oven and the convection oven is already discussed.

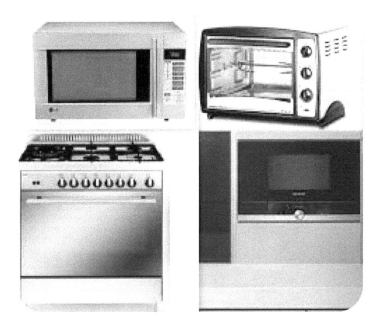

## 2.1 Culinary Ovens with Convection

The Convection ovens spread heat equally around the food. It enables food to cook more uniformly in much less time and at the lowest temperature compared to traditional oven. In 1914, the first oven with a fan to pump air was developed and commercially launched.

The Maxson Whirlwind is an Oven; developed in 1945; it was the first widely-used convection oven. This convection oven does have a ventilator in it along with a heating system. The air throughout the cooking area circulates through a tiny fan. As an insulator, the boundary layer of the hot air works and slows the pace at which the heat enters the food. The coating pushes the cold air away from the food, and cooking happens quicker. The heat is normally lowered by around 20 ° C (40 ° F) to depress overcooking until the center is baked. Furthermore, this oven does have a very consistent temperature, so the hot air is spread well. The Radiant heat points at the upper part and the lower part of the oven can be used in the convection ovens, improving heat transfer and cooking speeds from the preliminary cold start. On the other side, some ovens get all the heaters placed in an exterior framework and separated from food which eliminates the influence of the radiant heat on food. Furthermore, the escaping heated air will still heat the sides of the oven. The resultant heat is much lower than the heat generated from radiant heat source, however it is also hot enough to produce some heat from the walls to heat the food.

Compared to a traditional oven, a convection oven provides a decrease in the cooking temperature. The decrease in temperature depends on the conditions, for example, how much food is prepared at once or whether airflow is limited. The conditions may vary, for example, from an overloaded cooking tray. This variation in cooking temperature is compensated as heat is transferred more rapidly by the moving air than while air with the same temperature. To move the same volume of heat simultaneously and adjust; the heat must be reduced to minimize heat transfer intensity.

Product research has not proven that convection preparation in a toaster oven results in substantial toasting or baking benefits. However, air fryer, such as toaster ovens, which are larger toaster ovens with an incorporated convection fan element, has become very popular.

## 2.2 Other varieties of convection oven

The impingement oven is another kind of convection oven. This oven is mostly used in restaurants to bake pizzas and gently toast bread, but it may also be used elsewhere for foods other than this. Impingement ovens provide a strong hot air flow rate both from the up and down of the foods. The air movement is aimed at the food that normally moves on the conveyor belt. Impingement ovens may produce a much better heat transfer than just a traditional oven. Turbochef is the most popular producer of such a type of oven. Price, power usage, and pace difference between the impingement oven and the convection oven makes them distinct from one another. Impingement ovens are intended for use in restaurants, where pace is essential, and energy usage and expense are least concerned.

There are also convection microwave ovens that match the pace of a microwave oven to cook the food and match the convection oven's browning capacity. The air fryer is a simpler countertop oven that flows hot air through the oven. However, a higher degree of airflow is used for an air fryer. The combi steamer is also an oven that mixes overheated steam and convection technology to cook the food much quicker and preserve more nutrients and moisture.

## 2.3 Convection ovens for commercial applications

Commercial convection ovens may be very broad and are primarily used to manufacture multiple products at higher scale. We will not discuss them here because our main concern is to provide knowledge for consumers.

## 2.4. Convection ovens for customers

There are several distinct large and small convection ovens owned at consumer level. Some standard ovens arrive with an incorporated convection bake function, and others are mainly simple convection ovens. Many people have a simple convection oven, which is equivalent to the microwave or smaller and cooks stuff like beef, vegetables and even pizza. Some people have an air fryer that uses a tiny basket designed not to prepare entire meals but to reheat the frozen items.

The word "convection" is generally used to indicate "fan-assisted" in the sense of ovens. However, this is probably may not be the most appropriate way to discern fan-based ovens over traditional ovens, like all forms of oven work utilizing convection (heat transfer due to hot air bulk movement). Using the natural convection, traditional ovens circulate the hot air, and the fan-assisted ovens distribute the hot air using the artificial convection, so the word "convection" is scientifically applicable to both the conventional ovens and the fan-assisted ovens. Now that you have learned all about various convection ovens, we are now moving towards the answer to the most important question. When to and when not to use convection oven?

# Chapter 3: When and when not to use convection oven?

You are still curious that most of the convection ovens have a standard oven configuration when there are so many advantages to convection. There are times where you do not want a fan blowing hot air throughout, based on what you're making.

## 3.1 Why should the convection setting be used?

1. **It cooks faster:** When hot air blows directly on the food instead of only covering it, food cooks around 25 percent quicker then conventional oven.

2. **Uniform cooking of the food:** The fan in the convection oven can move the air to help balance out the temperature differences and avoid spotting on the food.

3. **Best browning:** The air will get a little sticky in a normal oven when the moisture can't getaway. Convection provides a dry environment. It caramelizes the sugars quicker, thus foods such as meats and vegetables become browner. However, the interiors remain moist.

4. **Energy effective:** Since food cooks better in convection oven, and normally at a low temp, it is a little more energy effective than a standard oven. It saves energy.

## 3.2 When to use the convection setting?

1. Roasting things, such as meats and vegetables is always best with convection setting. In this setting, they cook quicker, more consistently, and the drier atmosphere yields even crisps and caramelizes the outside of the skin.

2. Convection heat melts fat when baking pies and pastries and generates steam quicker, which helps to produce further lift in the pie doughs and pastries such as croissants.

3. Convection helps you bake uniformly over one tray of the cookies when there is no need to move them partway.

4. Whether you are covering the food with a plate, such as a braise, or cover the casserole dish in foil, when the lack of moisture is not a concern, then you should cook on convection, it will cook quicker.

5. When you toast or dehydrate: The aim is to extract moisture as easily as possible when you toast food. So, convection is more successful than normal in this case.

## 3.3 The Convection Configuration when not to be used

The fan becomes a burden for sensitive foods that begin as batter and held when cooking. It may produce lopsided outcomes by pumping air on such foods. When making these foods, don't use convection:

- Custards
- Flans
- Desserts
- Souffles
- Bread

**Loaves of bread:** Some people claim that convection also provides browning as well as a great crust, while other claim that the bread's interior dries out with convection setting. The decision now is up to you if you want to try baking bread or not.

## 3.4. How to utilize the Environment of Convection

Here are a few points to bear in mind if you want to use the convection setting:

1. **Lower the temperature:** Decrease the prescribed oven temperature by 25 ° F.

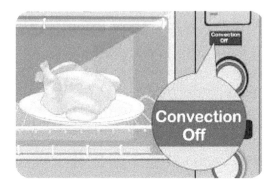

2. **Check earlier:** As food cooks on convection more rapidly, monitor it two-thirds to three-quarters and halfway into the prescribed cooking period and make any appropriate changes.

3. **Ensure the air must circulate:** The Convection is successful only if the air will move well through the food. Using lower-sided trays, the roasting pans and the baking pans do not line the oven shelf with foil.

Keep these points in mind and do not worry about the convection oven. Enjoy this wonderful function. Work around with it and the effects would certainly amaze you.

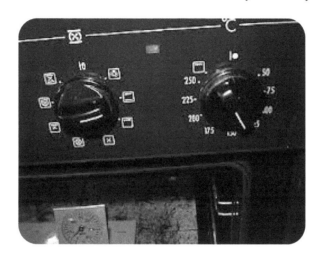

## 3.5 Drawbacks of convection oven

When it comes to baking, convection ovens have their disadvantages. The majority of convection ovens have a "bake" or the "thermal bake" feature that operates like a traditional oven. It is often safer to switch the convection fan off while baking since convection will cook the cake's exterior faster than the inside. The disparity in baking times can also be so pronounced that perhaps the top of the cake will flop over. When it's baked, the whole cake will dry out. Some bakers know how to work with the fans so that this doesn't happen, but for a daily chef, a ruined cake or two might cause them to hold the fans away entirely and switch to a traditional oven. Luckily, most convection ovens can switch off the fan. Fan speed can be changed in most convection ovens. High velocity is ideal for roasting, while low velocity is good for cookies and dehydration. You are still curious that most of the convection ovens do have a standard oven configuration when there are so many advantages to convection. There are times where you do not really want a fan blowing hot air throughout, based as to what you are making.

After learning answers to all the basic questions about convection oven, now you know all about the convection oven and ready to make some delicious recipes. So, let's start.

# Chapter 4: Convection Oven Chicken recipes

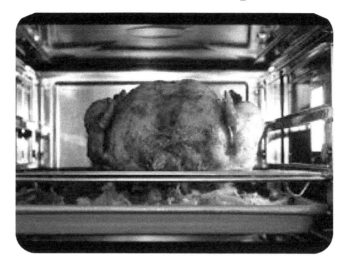

## 4.1 Chicken Broast

Preparation time: 1hr 20mins | Servings: 4 | Difficulty: Medium

**Ingredients**

- Chicken, whole 1
- Kosher salt, 3/4 tsp (teaspoon)
- Ground black pepper, 1/2 tsp
- Any fresh herb
- Garlic clove, 1 peeled
- Onion, 1 small
- Lemon zest of 4 slices of lemon
- Olive oil, 1 tbsp (tablespoon)
- Lemon juice, 1 tbsp

**Directions**

1. In the oven, put the toaster oven rack in the lowest spot. At the convection configuration, preheat the oven to 425 ° F.

2. Take the giblets and the neck from the chicken cavity, put aside for future usage, or dispose of. Rinse the chicken with cold water and wipe it dry.

3. In a broiling pan (which is lined by foil), put a baking rack, then add 1/4 cup of water to the pan and gently spray the baking rack with a cooking spray.

4. Now tuck the wings underneath and put the chicken in the tray over the baking rack. Disinfect the working surface and also hands with soap and the hot water.

5. Rub the herb sprig, the garlic halves, the onion quarters and the lemon zest on the chicken cavity.

6. Attach the legs loosely. Rub the olive oil and the remaining salt and the pepper on the chicken. Drizzle the lemon juice on it.

7. Put the chicken in the oven and cook for almost 20 minutes at 400 ° F, then reduce the temperature to 375 ° F and proceed to cook for another 12 minutes.

8. When examined in the breast, the chicken's internal temperature should be 170 ° F or 180 ° F.

9. Turn the oven off and put the chicken on a platter. Let stand 10 to 15 minutes until cutting (if desired, loosely cover with foil, but the skin may lack its crispness).

10. Bon Appetit.

## 4.2 Convection oven chicken wings

Preparation time: 1h 20mins | Servings: 24 wings | Difficulty: Medium

**Ingredients**

- Chicken wings, 4 lbs.
- Baking powder, 1 1/2 tbsp

- Seasoned salt, 1 tsp
- Garlic powder, 1 tsp
- Black pepper, 1/2 tsp
- Cayenne pepper, 1/4 tsp
- Butter melted, 3 tbsp.
- Buffalo sauce, 1/3 cup

**Directions**

1. Preheat the oven to 450 ° F temperature. Line a wide-rimmed baking sheet with foil, then put an oven-safe rack on its top. For non-stick spray, spritz and put aside.
2. To be sure that the chicken is dry, use lots of paper towels to get as much humidity out from the chicken wings as feasible.
3. In a wide bowl, mix some baking powder, the seasoned salt, black pepper, garlic powder and cayenne pepper and stir to combine. Rub it on chicken wings and coat equally with a flip.
4. On the prepared baking sheets, lay the chicken wings, making sure to give them space to not strike each other. Bake, then flip and bake for another 30 - 40 minutes until the chicken wings are crispy and golden.
5. In a big pan, now combine the melted butter with buffalo sauce, then whisk to combine. Rapidly toss the chicken wings into the sauce right before serving and eat afterward.
6. Bon Appetit.

## 4.3 Chicken and Potatoes Oven Roasted

Preparation time: 1h 20mins | Servings: 6 persons | Difficulty: Medium

**Ingredients**

Roasted Chicken

- Chicken, 1 whole

- Butter, 1/4 cup
- Italian dressing packet, 1 packet
- Garlic minced, 2 tsp
- Small lemon, 1/2

**Roasted Vegetables**

- Potatoes gold Yukon, 5-6 medium
- Carrots, 2-3 large
- Onion, 1 medium
- Avocado oil, 1 tbsp
- Garlic Salt, 1 tsp

**Directions**

1. To 400 °F, preheat the oven.

**Chicken Preparation**

1. Separate the giblets from the chicken. With a paper towel, pat the chicken dry. Put half a lemon into the chicken's cavity. With a string, bind the legs together and strap the wings under the chicken.
2. Now lightly salt and pepper the whole chicken.

**Preparation for Roasted Chicken Seasonings**

1. Apply the melted butter, the whole fine seasonings of Italian dressing package, and the minced garlic in the tiny mixing container.
2. Now utilize a fork and mix all of the ingredients.
3. Slather the butter mix all over the chicken using a fork, spoon or hand. (It's all right if it's a bit clumpy)

**How to Oven a whole chicken Roast**

1. In a glass baking bowl, place the chicken and put in the oven.

2. Wash the potatoes, the carrots, and onions and cut into 2-inch pieces, and transfer a tbsp of the cooking oil before putting it around the chicken. Scatter garlic and salt on vegetables.

3. Bake for 45 minutes in a 400 ° preheated oven. Check the chicken's internal temperature with the help of a meat thermometer. If the chicken's skin turns golden brown, then cover the chicken lightly with aluminum foil and proceed to bake till the chicken's internal temperature becomes 165 °. This cooking period is likely to be about 100-120 minutes.

4. Bring the chicken out from the oven for 5-10 minutes and let it cool. Serve and eat!

## 4.4 Baked simple Chicken Breasts

Preparation time: 1h 20mins | Servings: 4 persons | Difficulty: Medium

**Ingredients**

- Chicken breast halves, 4, skinless
- Olive oil, 2 tbsp s
- Coarse sea salt, 1 tbsp
- Creole seasoning, 1 pinch
- Water, 1 tbsp

**Directions**

1. Preheat the oven to the 400 ° F for convection.

2. With olive oil, brush the chicken breasts and then sprinkle with salt and the creole seasoning on both sides. Put the chicken in the broiler pan.

3. Now bake for 10 minutes within a preheated oven. Flip the chicken and cook till it is no longer raw in the middle, and the juices are transparent, around 15 more minutes. At least 165 ° F (74 ° C) can be readable via an immediate-read thermometer inserted into the core.

4. Take the chicken out from the pan.

5. Spill water into the pan by using a wooden spoon to clean the browned food scraps off the

container's bottom. If appropriate, apply more water to displace the browned scraps.

6. Now serve with chicken roast chicken and veggies.

## 4.5 Chicken veggie dish

Preparation time: 1h 5 min | Servings: 24 persons | Difficulty: Medium

**Ingredients**

- Chicken, 1 whole
- Grapeseed oil, ¼ cup
- Grapeseed oil, 1 tbsp
- Coarse salt, ½ tsp
- Pepper, ¼ tsp
- Cooking spray
- Red onion, 1 large
- Small potatoes, 1 lb.
- Carrots, 4 larges
- Fresh green beans, 1 cup

**Directions**

1. Rinse and pat dry the chicken, and then coat with a 1/4 cup of oil.
2. Now sprinkle some salt and pepper.
3. Now spray the bottom rack of the halogen cooker with the cooking spray.
4. Now place chicken's breast-side down on the rack.
5. Then cook at the temp of 350° for almost 30 minutes.
6. Lastly, take a large bowl, add veggies, some oil, a pinch of salt and pepper. Coat it now by flipping.

7. After some time is passed, turn the chicken over, now arrange the veggie around it, cook till the inner temperature of chicken breast is almost 165°.
8. Enjoy!

## 4.6 Lemon Garlic Roasted Chicken and Potato Wedges

Preparation time: 45 min | Servings: 4 persons | Difficulty: Medium

**Ingredients**

- Cut into pieces, 1 chicken.
- 2 lemon
- Potatoes, 3
- Olive oil, 1 tbsp
- Dried oregano, 1 tsp
- Garlic cloves 5
- Salt and ground pepper

**Directions**

1. Start by preheating the oven to 425° temperature.
2. Now toss the chicken with the ingredients except for the 1/2 of the lemon.
3. Then slice the 1/2 lemon and put it into the chicken and the potato mix.
4. Now place it on a roasting pan with chicken's skin up.
5. Lastly, cook at 425 convection for almost 45 minutes.
6. Check the doneness and then continue to cook another 10 min if required.
7. Serve.

## 4.7 Oven-Fried Extra Crispy Chicken Thighs

Preparation time: 35 min | Servings: 4 persons | Difficulty: Easy

**Ingredients**

- Chicken thighs, 10
- Baking powder, 1 tbsp
- Kosher salt, 2 tsp
- Sweet paprika, 2 tsp
- Black pepper, 1 tsp
- Sauce of Buffalo wing, 3 tbsp

**Directions**

1. Start by preheating the oven to 450F temperature.
2. First, dry the chicken thighs using some paper towels. Now sprinkle some salt, some paprika, pepper and the baking powder. Gently rub with the help of hands to ensure even coverage.
3. Then lay these chicken thighs on a cooking rack, parting a little space among pieces. Rub the rack with the oil to reduce sticking.
4. Bake for 25 min and serve.

## 4.8 Rotisserie styled chicken

Preparation time: 1 hr. 15 min | Servings: 6 servings | Difficulty: medium

**Ingredients**

- Paprika, 2 tbsp
- Dried thyme, 1 1/2 tbsp
- Garlic powder, 1 tsp
- Onion powder, 1 tsp

- Salt and ground black pepper
- Whole chicken, 1
- Olive oil, 1 tbsp s

**Directions**

**Chicken preparation**

1. Using a small bowl, mix paprika, some garlic powder, thyme onion powder, and as required, salt and pepper.
2. Now remove the giblets and then truss the chicken.

**Chicken in a rotisserie**

1. Truss the chicken.
2. Rub some spice mixture on the outer side of the chicken.
3. Put rotisserie skewers inside the rotisserie. Then cook according to the manufacturer's instructions.
4. Lastly, remove from the rotisserie and then allow to rest for 10 minutes.

**Chicken in oven**

1. First, move the oven rack to the lowest position. Preheat the oven to 425 °F.
2. Then place trussed chicken in the roasting pan.
3. Then brush the outside of the chicken with some olive oil. Rub some spice mixture on the chicken's outside area.
4. Now, bake it uncovered till the internal temperature ranges almost 165°, for about 70 - 80 minutes. Then take it out periodically and brush the chicken (for every 15-20 minutes) with juices accumulated beneath the dish to stop it from getting dry.
5. Then remove from the oven and allow to rest for 10 minutes before serving.
6. Serve.

## 4.9 Crispy convection Oven Baked Chicken Wings

Preparation time: 1 hour 15 minutes | Servings: 5 | Difficulty: medium

**Ingredients**

- Chicken wings, 18
- Flour, ½ cup
- Tony Chachere's seasoning, 1 tbsp
- Smoked paprika, ½ tsp
- Cooking spray

**Sauce**

- Barbecue sauce, 3/4 cup
- Honey, 1/2 cup
- Bourbon, 3 tbsps
- Chipotle in adobo, 1 tbsp
- Butter, 4 tbsps
- Garlic powder, 1/2 tsp

**Directions**

1. Start by preheating the oven to 425F temperature.
2. Now cover the baking sheet with the foil and then spray it with a cooking spray.

Bourbon Sauce preparation

1. Blend all the sauce ingredients.
2. Now simmer them on low heat, often stir, it becomes thick in almost 30 minutes.
3. Now turn the burner off and then let sauce cool while making wings. It will get thick.

Wings preparation

1. Split the wings and then separate the drums from the wings or let them leave as a whole.

2. Now blend the flour, the Tony Chachere's seasoning, along with some smoked paprika in a container.

3. Now blot the wings through a paper towel and dry it.

4. Dip the wings in the flour mixture till it thoroughly gets coated.

5. Next, arrange them in one layer on a baking sheet.

6. Place the baking sheet in the preheated oven.

7. Now cook for almost 15 minutes while watching carefully, don't burn.

8. Start turning the wings and then cook 20- 30 minutes. Keep on watching carefully.

9. Now remove it from the oven and then dip the wings into the sauce. Stay careful; they are hot.

10. Now place sauce-covered wings again back in the baking sheet.

11. Lastly, cook for almost 5 minutes or till an instant-read thermometer shows 160F-165F temperature.

12. Now remove from the oven and let it stand for 5 minutes.

13. Serve.

## 4.10 convection Baked Chicken Drumsticks

Preparation Time: 1 hour 5 minutes | Servings: 15 drumsticks | Difficulty: Easy

**Ingredients**

- Chicken drumsticks, 15
- Steve's BBQ rub, 1/3 cup.
- BBQ sauce, 1 cup

**Directions**

1. Start by preheating the oven to 400F.

2. Cover the chicken drumsticks in Steve's BBQ Rub. Now place them on a baking sheet which

is lined with parchment paper. Now make sure that drumsticks are not very close.

3. Bake for 30 minutes.

4. Take them out of the oven and brush them with half of the BBQ sauce. Now put back in the oven and bake for 15 minutes more.

5. Now take them out from the oven and start flipping the drumsticks. Then brush with the remaining BBQ sauce. Place back in the oven and bake almost 15 more minutes.

## 4.11 Baked Chicken Thighs Perfect Crispy

Preparation Time: 45 mins | Servings: 6 | Difficulty: medium

**Ingredients**

- Chicken thighs with skin, 2 lbs. bone-in
- Olive oil, 1 tbsp
- Onion powder, 1 tsp
- Garlic powder 1 tsp
- Pepper, 1/2 tsp
- Salt, 1/2 tsp
- Oregano, 1/2 tsp
- Basil, 1/2 tsp

**Directions**

1. Start heating the oven to 400°F temperature on the convection setting. Now line a rimmed baking sheet with the foil and also place a wire rack.

2. Now blot the chicken thighs with a paper towel till completely dry, now transfer to a large container.

3. Cover with oil till it gets thinly coated, and then transfer by keeping the skin side up.

4. Now stir together the rub, and then sprinkle over them on the thighs.

5. Now bake the chicken in the oven.

6. Check that the chicken is almost cooked through to reach the temperature of 165°F.

7. Allow them to rest for almost 5 minutes before serving.

8. Now serve.

## 4.12 Lemons and Garlic Roast Chicken

Preparation Time: 1 hr. 30 min | Servings: 4 | Difficulty: Medium

**Ingredients:**

- Chicken, 1
- Olive oil, 1 Tbs.
- Kosher salt and ground pepper
- 1 head garlic Clove
- Lemons halved, 3
- Fresh rosemary sprigs, 4

**Directions:**

1. Start by preheating the oven to 425°F.

2. Now rinse chicken inside out and then pat dry using paper towels. Now rub the chicken with some olive oil and then season it inside and outside with the salt and the pepper. Now place almost half of garlic cloves and lemon halves in the chicken cavity. Now tuck wing tips at the back and also tie the legs together.

3. Now put the chicken by keeping the breast side up, in a roasting pan. Then arrange rosemary sprigs, remaining garlic cloves, lemon halves over chicken. Then roast chicken till the skin is browned and an instant-read thermometer registers 170°F, 1 1/4 - 1 1/2 hours.

4. Now transfer chicken to a board, cover it loosely with an aluminum foil, and rest for almost 10 minutes. Now carve the chicken and then immediately with some roasted lemons and garlic alongside and pour the remaining juices from the pan.

## 4.13 Crispy Oven Chicken Tenders

Preparation time: 28 minutes | Servings: 4 | Difficulty: Medium

**Ingredients**

- Chicken breast tenders, 1 ½ pound
- Flour, ¼ cup
- Seasoned salt, ½ tsp
- Cornflake crumbs, 1 cup
- Panko breadcrumbs, 1 cup
- Garlic powder, ½ tsp
- Paprika, 1 tsp
- Pepper and salt
- Eggs beat, 2

**Directions**

1. Start by preheating the oven to 425°F temperature. Now line the pan with parchment paper.
2. Now cut the chicken breasts into pieces of size 3/4" pieces.
3. Put the flour and the seasoned salt in the bowl.
4. Now add cornflake crumbs, garlic powder, panko breadcrumbs, and salt and pepper along with paprika to taste.
5. Now lightly dredge the chicken in the flour, dip them in eggs, and finally dip them in the bread crumb mix.
6. Finally, place chicken on the prepared pan and then spray with a cooking spray.
7. Now bake for 18-22 minutes till it is cooked thoroughly.

## 4.14 Roasted Chicken with Lemon Garlic flavored Potato Wedges

Preparation time: 30 minutes | Servings: 4 | Difficulty: Easy

**Ingredients**

- Orange juice, 2 tbsp
- Soy sauce, 5 tbsp
- Thai chili sauce, 5 tbsp
- Garlic powder ,1 tsp
- Sesame oil, 1tsp
- Seasoned rice vinegar, 5 tbsp
- Asparagus spears, 12 thin.
- Green onion, chopped, 2 tbsp
- Chicken, 1

**Directions**

1. Start by preheating the oven to 450 °F. Put the first six ingredients in the bowl.
2. Now tear them off in a 12x18 inch heavy foil. Now fold it in half lengthwise with the dull side within.
3. Then spray the dull side with the cooking spray. Place the chicken on one side of the foil and then cut the chicken into half with the knife. Pour sauce on chicken, then pile vegetables on top.
4. Fold top and sides of the foil close and place on a cookie sheet. Bake 15-20 minutes.
5. Serve

## 4.15 Pepper chicken with potato wedges

Preparation time: 60 minutes | Servings: 4 | Difficulty: Medium

**Ingredients**

- Chicken, 1
- Lemons, 2
- Potatoes, 2 cut into wedges.
- Olive oil, 1 tbsp
- Dried oregano, 1 tsp
- Garlic cloves, 5
- Salt and pepper

**Directions**

1. Start by preheating the oven to 425 °F temperature in a convection oven.
2. Now toss chicken with ingredients.
3. Then slice almost 1/2 lemon and then put it into the chicken and the potato mix.
4. Now place in roasting pan chicken by keeping the skin up. Cook at 425 for almost 45 minutes and check doneness. Continue to cook for another 10 minutes.
5. Serve.

## 4.16 Golden Roast Hens with delicious vegetable hash

Preparation time: 60 minutes | Servings: 4 | Difficulty: Medium

**Ingredients**

- Cornish hens, 2
- Balsamic vinegar, ¼ cup

- Olive oil, 3 tbsp
- Soy sauce, 2 tbsp
- Sage leaves, 1 tbsp
- Garlic, 2 cloves
- Banana squash, 1 piece
- Yukon Gold potato, 1
- Red bell pepper, 1
- Onion, 1
- Sage leaves, 6 freshes
- Salt, 1/4 tsp
- Pepper, 1/8 tsp

**Directions**

1. Remove the necks and the giblets from the hens and reserve. Now rinse the hens and then pat them dry. In a 1-gallon plastic bag, put vinegar, olive oil, some soy sauce, chopped sage, and garlic. Now add hens. Then seal the bag and let it chill, turn it occasionally, up to one day.

2. Then rinse the squash, potato, and bell pepper. Cut and discard the skin from the squash. Peel the onion. Cut the squash, pepper, potato, and onion into pieces of 1/2-inch; now put them in the 9/ 13-inch sized baking pan. Transfer the remaining two tbsps olive oil and remaining garlic, whole sage leaves, salt, and pepper, and then mix well.

3. Now lift the hens from the marinade, and discard the marinade. Place the chicken on a rack in 10- 15-inch sized baking pan. Now tie the ends of the drumsticks slightly together with a cotton string.

4. Place the vegetables on the top rack and then hens on the bottom rack for a 425° temperature in a convection oven. Now roast and stir vegetables until vegetables become browned and tender after being pierced, for about 45 - 60 minutes.

5. Now add some salt and some pepper to the hash as needed. Then transfer in the plates/platter. Now arrange chicken alongside.

# Chapter 5: Beef and lamb

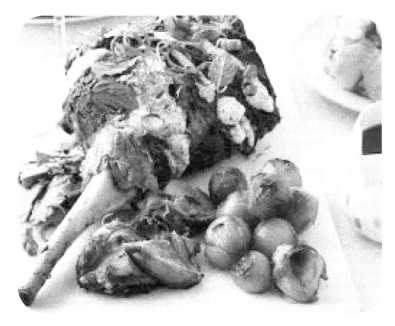

## 5.1. Prime Rib

Preparation time: 1 hr. 45 min | Servings: 8 | Difficulty: Medium

**Ingredients**

- Prime Rib Roast, 1
- Butter, 1 tbsp
- Salt and pepper, to taste

**Directions**

1. Roasts cooked in the convection ovens can be up to 30 ° higher internally compared to roasts cooked in standard ovens. If you want your roast to turn out evenly, use a meat thermometer to determine its internal temperature rather than the period it has been cooking.

2. Cut fat from both sides of the prime rib in a total of 1 inch and enable it to remain loosely

covered till it has hit room temperature — approximately 2 hours after bringing it outside the refrigerator.

3. With a paper towel, drain it, then pat it dry. Slather with salt and pepper and put it in a deep roasting pan, which will match inside the convection oven. Sprinkle butter all across cut edges. Do not use nonstick pans as its surface leaches toxic chemicals into the braising liquid.

4. Within convection oven, set at the optimum temperature (around 450 ° F), put the rib with fatty side up, about 15 minutes, after which turn down the heat to 325 ° F., inspect and braise it every 1/2 hour.

5. Around 1/2 hour well before the expected end of the roasting period, monitor the roast via an interior meat thermometer.

6. When it hits 110 ° F, put a meat thermometer then extract it. Keep it to 125 ° F m medium for doneness.

7. Until eating, enable the roasted rib to sit for at least 20 minutes. The core temperature will remain hot throughout that time, and the juices would be trapped in the meat. The roast will continue to cook, but don't let it stay for too long.

8. Serve.

## 5.2. Honey Pork Chops Grilled

Preparation time: 50 min | Servings: 6 | Difficulty: Easy

**Ingredients**

- Ketchup, ½ cup
- Honey, 2 ⅔ tbsp
- Soy sauce, 2 tbsps
- Crushed, 2 cloves garlic
- Dried chilies, 1 tsp

- Pork chops, trimmed 6

**Directions**

1. First, spray the rack of a convection oven with some cooking Spray.
2. Now set the oven at the temperature of 225°F.
3. Then, whisk ketchup, garlic, honey, and soy sauce together in the bowl to make a coating.
4. Now lightly brush the glaze all around the chops.
5. Now, arrange chops on the rack of the oven and cook for about 30 minutes.
6. Lastly, turn chops over, brush chops with some glaze again and then cook until the chops turn crispy
7. Serve.

## 5.3. Sicilian-style Strata

Preparation time: 50 min | Servings: 6 | Difficulty: Medium

**Ingredients**

- Italian-style bread, 1 loaf crusty
- Prosciutto or ham slices
- Red peppers, diced 1/4 cup
- Sliced green onions, 1/4 cup
- Grated parmesan cheese, 1/2 cup
- Chopped tomatoes, 1 can
- Pitted black olives, 1/4 cup
- Shredded mozzarella, 1/2 cup
- Eggs, 6 larges
- Milk, 3 cups

- Dried Italian seasoning, 2 tbsp
- Salt, 1/2 tsp
- Pepper, 1/2 tsp
- Chopped parsley, 1/4 cup
- Drained capers, 2 tbsps

**Directions**

1. First, spread almost half of the bread cubes and level in the lightly oiled baking pan. Then top evenly with some prosciutto, parmesan cheese, peppers, green onions. Next, spread the remaining bread cubes on the top, followed by some tomatoes, mozzarella and olives.
2. Whisk eggs, salt, and pepper, milk, Italian seasoning in a bowl to blend. Then pour it over the layered ingredients. Next, cover it and then chill for at least 1 hour for one day.
3. Lastly, bake in 325° convection oven until the strata center is almost set and the top is browned lightly, for 40 - 50 minutes.
4. Now sprinkle with parsley and some capers. Then let it stand for 10 minutes and then cut them into squares.
5. Now serve them warm.

## 5.4. South-west Cheese Puff Pot Beef Pie

Preparation time: 50 min | Servings: 6 | Difficulty: Easy

**Ingredients**

- Puff pastry sheet, 1 frozen
- Milk, 2 tbsps
- Shredded cheddar cheese, ⅓ cup
- Zucchini, 3
- Onion, 1

- Canned chipotle chilies, 2 to 4
- Cumin seed, 1 tsp
- Olive oil, 1 tsp
- Stewed tomatoes, 2 cans
- Yellow hominy, 1 can
- Beef pot roast and gravy, 1 package
- Cornstarch, 2 tbsps
- Salt and pepper, as needed.

**Directions**

1. Unfold the pastry on the board, gently flour. Rollover or cut the pastry to accommodate the shallow 3-quart casserole snugly within the end. Move the pastry to the non-stick baking sheet, which is 12 x 15 inches. To produce a decorative shape, break through the pastry in many locations. Brush with milk gently and scatter with cheese uniformly. Wrap up and freeze with plastic wrap on it.

2. Cut them into 3/4-inch parts, drain the zucchini, then trim and discard the ends. Peel and slice the onion into 3/4-inch chunks. Discard the stems of chipotle chili and remove veins and the seeds. Chop the chilies.

3. Uncover the pastry and cook until they are golden brown, 15 - 20 minutes, in a 425 ° convection oven.

4. Meanwhile, mix the zucchini, onion, & cumin in the olive oil continuously in a 5 x 6-quart pan on high heat till the vegetables become nicely browned, 7–9 minutes. Stir in tomatoes, juice included, and the hominy; bring to a simmer.

5. Discard some fat and the sauce from the pot roast. Scrape with beef gravy and then reserve. Break the beef into almost 3/4-inch bits.

6. Combine, incorporate beef and gravy in the pan; cover and bring to the boil. Reduce to low heat and cook, stirring regularly, 7–9 minutes, till the beef is hot. For sample purposes,

apply the chilies. Mix the cornstarch with three tbsps of water in a shallow bowl. Transfer to the saucepan and whisk until the mixture cooks.

7. In a heated, shallow casserole, dump the hot mixture into it. Place the hot pastry onto the filling. To smash through the pastry and scoop out the portions, use a large spoon.

8. Serve.

## 5.5. Meatloaf

Preparation time: 1 hr. 30 min | Servings: 6-8 | Difficulty: Medium

**Ingredients**

- Breadcrumbs, 1 cup fresh
- Milk, 1/3 cup
- Ground chuck, 1 1/2 pounds
- Ground pork, 1/2 pound
- Butter, 2 tbsps
- Onion, diced 2 larges.
- Celery stalks, diced 2
- Carrot, diced, 1 medium
- Cloves, minced, 2 garlic
- Creme fraiche, 1/2 cup
- 2 eggs, beaten
- Worcestershire sauce, 2 tbsp
- Dry mustard powder, 1 tsp
- Paprika, 1 tsp
- Fresh parsley, chopped, 2 tbsps
- Kosher salt, 1 1/2 tbsp

- Freshly black pepper, 1 tsp
- Slices bacon, 6
- Ketchup, 1 cup
- Brown sugar, 2 tbsps
- Dijon mustard, 1 tbsp
- Freshly grated nutmeg, 1/4 tsp

**Directions**

1. Preheat the oven to about 350 º F. Place the breadcrumbs in a small bowl and then drizzle the milk. Just set it aside.

2. In a broad pan, heat the butter and include the onion, celery & carrot. Slather with a pinch of salt and bake until the vegetables are juicy but not fully cooked, stirring periodically. Add garlic and then cook 2-3 more minutes. Take out from heat, dump it into a small bowl, and cool (approximately 10 minutes) at room temperature.

3. In another bowl, mix all the beaten eggs, the creme fraiche and the Worcestershire sauce.

4. Transfer the breadcrumb mix, vegetables, the egg mixture, and the remainder of the ingredients, excluding the bacon, brown sugar, ketchup, and mustard, to a big bowl of beef and pork. Use the hands to blend the meatloaf and ingredients thoroughly and put them inside a large oven-safe baking dish. Position five slices of bacon over meatloaf lengthwise; cut the remaining slice of bacon in half and put at the end of the loaf.

5. Set the alarm for 45 minutes and place it in the oven. In the meantime, mix and set aside ketchup, brown sugar, mustard and nutmeg. Preheat the oven to convection after 45 minutes and bake the meatloaf for a further 15 minutes. Take the meatloaf from of the oven when done and drop or spray glaze all around the bacon surface (it's okay if any splashes down into the pan). Put it back in and bake before the glaze bubbles for an extra 15 minutes. Take it out of the oven and let it rest for fifteen min.

6. Serve.

## 5.6 Easy Calzone

Preparation time: 1 hr. 30 min | Servings: 6-8 | Difficulty: Medium

### Ingredients

- Ground beef, 3/4 pound
- Chopped onion, 1/2 cup
- Pizza sauce, 1 can
- Dried basil, 1/2 tsp
- Dried oregano, 1/2 tsp
- Hoagie rolls, 4
- Shredded part-skim, 1-1/2 cups, mozzarella cheese

### Directions

1. Cook the beef and the onions over medium heat skillet until the meat isn't any longer pink, and rinse. Stir in pizza sauce, basil, and some oregano; boil for five minutes.
2. In the meantime, cut each roll 1/2 inch longitudinally from the tops; set the tops aside from the end. Roll them from sides and bottom. Sprinkle each roll with 3 tbsps of cheese: spoon meat sauce uniformly over the rolls. Slather with the cheese that remains.
3. In foil, cover each roll individually. Bake at 375 ° or till heated.
4. Serve hot.

## 5.7 Meatballs

Preparation time: 57 min | Servings: 30 balls | Difficulty: Medium

### Ingredients

- Beef, 8 oz ground
- Ground pork, 8 oz
- Yellow onion, 1/2 medium

- Garlic cloves, minced, 3
- Italian parsley, 1/4 cup, finely chopped
- Unseasoned panko, 1/2 cup breadcrumbs
- Grated Parmesan cheese, 1/4 cup
- Egg, 1
- Kosher salt, 1/2 tsp
- Ground pepper, 1/2 tsp

**Directions**

1. Combine all the components, then cover and leave to sit for 30 minutes.
2. Preheat oven to 350 ° F for convection cooking for 15 minutes only with rack in the center spot.
3. Spray with cooking spray on a large sheet of the pan and let it stand. Shape the mix into balls with a diameter of around 1 inch and put on the shelf. Sprinkle all the meatballs gently with the cooking spray.
4. Bake, once done, for 15 minutes.
5. Position the pan with meatballs roughly 4" from its broiler element to toast the meatballs and put the oven settings on "Broil." Watch carefully for the desired browning period (cook for 1 minute) and withdraw it from the oven.
6. Serve

## 5.8 Prosciutto Roast Pork Tenderloin

Preparation time: 1 hr. 30 min | Servings: 6-8 | Difficulty: Medium

**Ingredients:**

- Pork tenderloins, 2
- Prosciutto, 12 sheets
- Thyme, finely diced, 1 tbsp.
- Lemon zest, 1 tbsp.
- Olive oil, 2 tbsp
- Apples, 4 smalls
- Fennel, 1 bulb
- Feta cheese, 1/3 cup
- Shelled raw pistachios, 1/3 cup
- Parsley, 1/2 cup
- Honey, 1 tbsp

**Directions**

1. On a cutting board, put your pork and extract any extra fat. Spray the tenderloins with about one tbsp of the olive oil and then roll in the thyme and lemon zest.

2. Around each tenderloin, wrap six strips of prosciutto, surrounding the meat. Securely bind five or six pieces of butcher's twine across the meat to guarantee that the prosciutto remains along with the pork. Put the baking sheet with sides in the middle.

3. Halve the apples and put them in a bowl. Then top and tail the fennel bulb and then dice into strips, apply to the apples. Season it with a slight sprinkle of salt and some pepper. With 1 tsp of olive oil, mix the apples and the fennel. With both the apples and fennel, cover the outside of the baking tray.

4. Mount one of the tenderloins with the thermometer so that the tip lies within the middle of the beef's thickest portion. Insert the device's connection end into the thermometer's container, positioned from the oven cavity wall upon the upper left. Push the plus key to adjust

the temperature of the meter to 155 °.

5. Pick convection Bake and adjust to 425 ° F.

6. Put the baking tray within the oven and bake till the temperature measures 155 °, around 20 to 25 minutes. Extract and wrap for 10-15 minutes lightly within the aluminum foil.

7. Sprinkle the whole tray with one tbsp of honey and cover it with pistachios, parsley, and feta.

8. Serve.

## 5.9 Perfect Beef Jerky

Preparation time: 45 min | Servings: 6-8 | Difficulty: Medium

**Ingredients**

- Beef round, 2 pounds 1/8-inch strips
- Worcestershire sauce, 1 cup
- Soy sauce, 1 cup
- Brown sugar, 1 cup
- Liquid smoke, 1 tbsp
- Onion powder, 1 tbsp
- Garlic powder, 1 tbsp
- Black pepper, 1 tbsp
- Chili powder, 1 tsp
- Pepper flakes, 1 tsp

**Directions**

1. Transfer the steak strips to ziplock bag.
2. In a mixing bowl, whisk the remaining ingredients until combined. Pour mixture in the ziplock bag, seal the bag, and evenly coat the strips.

3. Refrigerate for 30 minutes.

4. Heat oven to 175°F. Adjust racks to upper and lower-middle location. Line 2 large baking sheets with foil and place it in wire racks. Lay the strips in single layer on the racks. Bake until it is dry for about 4 hours. Flip it once about halfway through.

5. Transfer to sealed container.

6. Refrigerate for almost a month.

## 5.10. Roast Leg of Lamb with Herbs

Preparation time: 2 hr. s | Servings: 8 | Difficulty: Medium

**Ingredients**

- Lamb, 1 leg
- Dry white wine, 3 tbsps of lemon juice
- Chopped parsley, 2 tbsps
- Chopped mint leaves, 2 Tbsps
- Olive oil, 2 tbsp
- Minced garlic, 1 tbsp
- Paprika, 1 tsp
- Crushed dried bay leaves, 1/2 tsp
- Pepper, 1/2 tsp
- Salt as desired

**Directions**

1. Dry lamb and pat rinse; skim off then and discard extra fat.

2. Combine vinegar, olive oil, garlic, parsley, mint, paprika, bay leaves, with 1/2 tsp pepper inside a shallow bowl. Brush the lamb all across.

3. Put the lamb in an 11 x 17-inch tray on the rack. Roast in a normal or convection oven at

375 ° till a thermometer placed into bone thru the thickest section of meat measures 140 ° under medium-rare, around 1 1/2 hours, or measures 150 ° for medium, around 1 3/4 hrs. If juices begin to burn, add water into the pan, as required, 1/4 cup at one time.

4. Move lamb to just a rimmed board/ platter and let stand for 10 minutes, holding it warm.

    Slice meat and serve from the bone. Apply salt to taste. 4. Move lamb to just a rimmed board/ platter and let stand for 10 minutes, holding it warm. Slice meat and serve from the bone. Apply salt to taste.

5. Serve.

## 5.11. Lamb Shanks with Olives and Capers

Preparation time: 1 hr. 30 min | Servings: 6 | Difficulty: Medium

**Ingredients**

- Lamb shanks, 6
- Capers, drained, 1 jar
- Pitted green olives 1 1/2 cups in brine
- Fresh rosemary leaves, 1/4 cup of dried rosemary, 3 tbsps
- Dry white wine, 1 bottle
- Fresh-ground pepper, 2 tbsp
- Grated lemon peel, 2 tbsp
- Lemon juice, 3 tbsps
- Lemon couscous
- Watercress sprigs, about 3 cups, rinsed and crisped

**Directions**

1. Rinse the lamb and pat dry it; lay shanks beside each other in a pan around 2 inches deep

inside a 12 x17-inch pan. Bake in a normal or convection oven at 450°, rotating once, around 25 minutes overall until the meat is very well browned. Decrease the temperature of the oven to 325°.

2. Meanwhile, put capers, olives in the fine strainer, rinse with cold water, and drain. Mince rosemary and combine in the blender with about 1 cup of the wine and mix until minced. Sprinkle capers, some olives, and rosemary onto lamb (or pour uniformly over the lamb rosemary-wine blend), apply the wine, stir it around shanks and scrape off browned pieces. Sprinkle the wine.

3. Bake for 3 to 3 1/4 hours until the meat is soft once pierced but pulls quickly from the bone.

4. Spoon into large, shallow bowls equivalent amounts of Lemon Couscous. Take lamb shanks from the pan with tongs and put one from each bowl on couscous. Trim and remove fat off pan juices. Ladle juices over meat with the olives and the capers. Then garnish the bowl with around 1/2 cup sprigs of watercress.

5. Serve.

## 5.12. Roast Beef

Preparation time: 1 hr. 30 min | Servings: 6-8 | Difficulty: Medium

**Ingredients**

- Beef rump roast, 2 1/2 - 3 lbs.
- Olive oil, 1 tbsp
- Garlic, 3 cloves
- Kosher salt
- Black pepper, freshly cracked

**Directions**

1. Take roast out from the refrigerator and thaw at room temperature. To 375 °F, preheat the

oven. Create a tiny slit in the meat only big enough for a sharp knife to slip a tiny piece of garlic into the meat. Repeat all around the roast, with each garlic piece. Drizzle the roast with olive oil, then rub it all over the edges. Sprinkle in salt and pepper over the whole roast. Position the roast immediately upon this oven rack, fatty side up, on even a rack beneath the roasting rack with a drip pan.

2. For 30 minutes, brown the roast at 375 º F. Adjust the heat to 225 F. Cook your roast for an extra 2-3 hours. Test the temperature with a meat thermometer as the roast starts to spill juices but has changed color on the outside. When the interior temperature is 140 F, gently use tongs to separate the roast from the oven. Just let roast rest on a plate to stay warm, tented with foil, with at least 15 minutes to serve before carving.

3. Enjoy.

# Chapter 6: Desserts

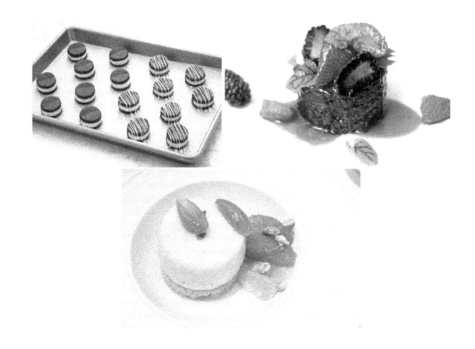

## 6.1. Convection Spooky Cake

Preparation Time: 45 | Servings: 6 | Difficulty: Easy

**Ingredients**

- Dark chocolate cake mixes, 1 box
- Eggs, 3 larges
- Oil, 1/3 cup
- Water, 1 cup
- White cake mixture, 1 box
- Egg whites, 3 larges

- Oil, ¼ cup
- Water, 1 cup

Ganache:

- Dark chocolate chips, 9 oz
- Whipping cream, 1 cup
- For drizzle orange ganache
- Orange chocolate, ½ cup
- Heavy cream, ¼ cup

**Directions**

1. Blend the chocolate cake mix with eggs, water, and oil as per box instructions; set aside the batter. Prepare a white cake mix in a medium bowl with egg whites, the oil and the water as per the package instructions.

2. Drop two scoops of white cake batter into the bundt cake dish, utilizing an ice cream scooper. Then, add 2 scoops of white chocolate batter in the end. Continue to turn between white and chocolate batters before you fill the Bundt pan.

3. Bake in the convection oven according to instructions from the package. Cool and transfer it from the pan to the cooling rack as directed.

4. **Chocolate Ganache:** In a medium bowl, insert the chocolate chips. Over medium boil heats the cream in a shallow saucepan. Simmer, and watch very closely since it can boil out from the pot.

5. Pour it out on chopped chocolate when the cream has come to simmer, then stir until smooth. If needed, stir in a touch of rum. Before pouring over the cake, enable the ganache to cool slowly.

6. Begin in the middle of the cake and push towards the outside.

7. Enable the mixture to settle until thick.

8. Enjoy.

## 6.2. Brie Filo-wrapped

Preparation Time: 45 minutes | Servings: 8 | Difficulty: Medium

**Ingredients**

- Dried tomatoes 1/4 cup
- Melted butter 2 tbsps
- Filo dough 4 sheets
- Basil leaves 1/4 cup fresh chopped.
- Brie cheese 1 round
- Pine nuts 1/4 cup

**Directions**

1. Put the nuts in a 9-inch pan for pie and bake until crispy, (5- 7 minutes), in a 350 ° standard or a convection oven.
2. In the meantime, chop the tomatoes. Blend the oil and the butter in a shallow container.
3. Cut the sheets of the filo into 12-inch squares. Brush squares gently one by one with some butter mixture and a stack.
4. Spread sliced tomatoes, basil, and some toasted nuts in the middle of a filo stack. Set the cheese on top of the mixture of tomatoes. Fold the filo corners, one by one, over the cheese, then gently brush with the butter mixture. To make it smooth, push the filo against the cheese.
5. Put the wrapped cheese inside a 9-inch pie pan, smooth the side up. Then brush with the remaining butter mixture on the top of the filo.
6. Now bake in a standard 350 ° or the convection oven for 25 to 30 minutes until the filo turns golden. Now cool for ten minutes.
7. Switch the wrapped filo brie to a plate using a large spatula. Cut a wide X in the middle or

cut apart a corner to offer so that that guest can spoon out the cheese mixture.

## 6.3. Choco Nut Brownies

Preparation Time: 40 minutes | Servings: 12 | Difficulty: Easy

**Ingredients**

- Unsalted butter, 1/2 cup
- Unsweetened chocolate, 2 ounces
- Sugar, 1 cup
- 2 eggs
- Vanilla, 1 tsp
- Unbleached flour, 2/3 cup
- Chopped nuts, 1/2 cup
- Baking powder, 1/2 tsp
- Salt ¼ tsp

**Directions**

1. Heat the convection oven to 350 ° C. -Grease and gently flour 8 9-inch square sheet base.
2. Melt the butter & chocolate on low heat in a big saucepan, stir continuously.
3. Remove from the heat; mildly cold. Blend with sugar. Whisk in the eggs, one by one. Stir the remaining components together. Place in a ready-made plate. Bake for 25- 30 minutes at 350 ° F until it's set in the middle.
4. If you like a lighter center, become careful not to overbake. Pull from the oven and cool on a wire rack entirely. Split into serving bars.

# 6.4 Chocolate chip cookies

Preparation Time: 30 minutes | Servings: 12 | Difficulty: Easy

**Ingredients**

- All-purpose flour, 1 cup
- Grated jaggery, 1/2 cup
- Caster sugar, 1/2 cup
- Baking powder, 1 tsp
- Baking soda, 1/2 tsp
- Salt, 1/4 tsp
- Melted butter, 1/4 cup
- Butter, 1/2 tsp
- 1 egg
- Vanilla essence, 1 tsp
- Dark chocolate, 1/2 cup chopped.

**Directions**

1. Sieve together the flour, baking powder, baking soda & some salt and leave this dried mixture aside.
2. Then, place melted butter in a big bowl and transfer the egg to it.
3. Drop the jaggery, the caster sugar and essence of vanilla.
4. Till the mixture is very smooth and lumps free, blend it very well.
5. Then add your dry mixture to the wet mixture little by little and blend it well till the cookie dough is prepared.
6. Apply the sliced dark chocolate to both the cookie dough and blend it up.
7. Grease a butter-based baking tray.

8. Take a few small bits of the cookie dough and place them on the greased tray, about 1 inch across each cookie dough.

9. Place the tray in the preheated microwave for 10 minutes in convection mode at 200 ° C and bake cookies for eight minutes at 180 ° C.

10. Remove the tray when the cookies are ready and just let cookies cool completely

11. Eventually, serve with some hot milk or coffee cookies.

## 6.5 Christmas Magic Bars

Preparation Time: 45 minutes | Servings: 25 | Difficulty: Easy

**Ingredients**

- Salted butter, 1/3 cup
- Baking crumbs, 1 1/2 cups
- Condensed milk, 300ml can
- Flaked coconut, 1 1/2 cups
- Red and green cherries chopped, 1 cup
- Chocolate chips, 1 cup

**Direction**

1. Heat the oven to 350 ° F in advance.
2. In an 8x8 tray apply the butter. For quicker removal, line the pan with tinfoil.
3. In an even layer, scatter the cookie crumbs on the top of the butter.
4. Transfer some condensed milk from the spoonful onto the crumbs, making an even layer.
5. Drizzle the three remaining ingredients over condensed milk in the order specified. Gently press down.
6. Bake in the oven till it becomes browned for 25 to30 minutes.
7. Cut and cool fully in the skillet. Use the tinfoil to remove it and carve it out.

## 6.6 Creme Brule

Preparation Time: 1 hr. | Servings: 12 | Difficulty: Easy

**Ingredients**

- Egg yolks, 6
- Cups sugar, 3
- Cream, 32 ounces
- Vanilla bean, 1
- Turbinado sugar

**Directions**

1. Heat the cream until warm, on medium heat.
2. Mix the eggs and sugar with milk and whisk together until the paste is white.
3. Slowly whisk the cream, make sure that the eggs are not scrambled.
4. Pour in ramekins, place in the oven within the water bath, bake for 45 minutes at a temperature of 325 ° F.
5. Sprinkle with Turbinado sugar
6. Serve.

## 6.7 Olive Oil Granola with cherries and pecans

Preparation time: 15 mins | Servings: 12 | Difficulty: Easy

**Ingredients**

- Rolled oats, 3 cups
- Raw pecan, 1 cup halves
- Sliced, raw almonds 3/4 cup
- Pumpkin seeds, 1/2 cup

- Sweetened coconut, 1/2 cup
- Sesame seeds, 1/4 cup
- 3/4 cup, dried cherries
- Maple syrup, 3/4 cup
- Vanilla, 1/2 tsp.
- Olive oil, 1/2 cup
- Brown sugar, 1/4 cup
- Kosher salt, 1 tsp.
- Cinnamon, 1/2 tsp.
- Cardamom, 1/2 tsp.

**Directions**

1. Preheat the 275-convection oven or 300 F for the regular or convection oven. Mix all ingredients together in a wide bowl except for the cherries and then spoon out onto a wide, rimmed baking dish. Bake till browned.
2. Serve.

## 6.8. Gingersnap Baked Apples

Preparation time: 1 hr. | Servings: 8 | Difficulty: Easy

**Ingredients**

- Gingersnap cookies, 3 ounces
- Brown sugar, 2 tbsps
- Apples, 4 sweet
- Butter rinsed, 1/4 cup.
- Whipping cream, 1/2 cup

**Directions**

1. Mix Gingersnaps and brown sugar into small crumbs in the mixer or the food processor.

2. Cut the apples around cores up to around 3/4 with a thin, sharp knife, beginning from stem ends; pick out cores with the spoon, creating a 1 1/2-inch-wide cavity and then keeping bases unaffected. In the shallow 2 3-quart baking dish, set the apples moderately apart.

3. Spoon each cavity with 1 tbsp of ginger snap mixture and finish with 1/2 tbsp of butter. Sprinkle the apples generously with the remaining blend of ginger.

4. Bake in a standard or convection oven of 375o until apples are soft, around 45 minutes until pierced. Shift into individual bowls and, if necessary, pour 2 tbsp of cream around each.

5. Serve

## 6.9 Pear and Ginger Cake

Preparation time: 45 mins | Servings: 4 | Difficulty: Medium

**Ingredients**

- Butter, 1/2 cup
- Brown sugar, 1 1/2 cups
- Crystallized ginger, 3 tbsps
- Bosc pears, 2 firm-ripe
- All-purpose flour, 2 1/2 cups
- Baking powder, 2 tbsp
- Baking soda, 1 tsp
- Ground ginger, 1 1/2 tbsp
- Ground cinnamon, 1 tsp
- Salt, 1/2 tsp
- Ground all spice, 1/4 tsp

- Eggs, 2 larges

- Dark molasses, 3/4 cup

- Buttermilk, 1 1/4 cups

**Directions**

1. Start by lightly buttering a 9-inch cake pan with a removable rim measuring 2 1/2 inches in height. Now line pan with a 10-inch round of cooking parchment paper, pressing the bottom and then 1/2 inches upsides. Then cut 2 tbsps of butter into the 1/4-inch chunks, drop them evenly over the parchment in the pan bottom. Sprinkle them evenly with a 1/2 cup of brown sugar and also with crystallized ginger.

2. Now peel pears and then cut in half lengthwise, afterward slicing them parallel to cut the edge, cut them into 1/2-inches thick slices. Now with the help of a small knife, tear core from all slices. Now arrange the slices flat, into a single layer, place over the sugar mixture in the pan, then trim the pieces as needed.

3. Whisk in a small bowl, some flour, baking soda, ginger, baking powder, cinnamon, salt, and spices.

4. With the help of an electric mixer, beat together the remaining 1/2 cup of butter and 1 cup of brown sugar until well blended in another bowl. Now add eggs and beat well. Then reduce the speed of the blender to medium-low and then beat in the molasses. Now add the flour mixture and the buttermilk alternately, beat until combined, and then beat again on high speed until well blended. Now pour the batter over the pears.

5. Now bake in 325° convection oven till the toothpick inserted in the center of the cake comes out clean, for 1 hour 35 minutes. Let it cool in the pan on the rack for about 20 min. Now remove the pan sides. Now invert the platter over the cake, hold the two together, then invert again. Now carefully remove the pan bottom and also the parchment.

6. Serve.

## 6.10. Louisiana Pecan Balls

Preparation time: 45 min | Servings: 28 cookies | Difficulty: Medium

**Ingredients**

- Butter, 1 cup
- Powdered sugar, 2 cups
- Vanilla, 2 tbsp
- All-purpose flour, 2 cups
- Baking powder, 1/4 tsp
- Chopped pecans, 1 cup

**Directions**

1. With the help of a mixer on a medium speed, start beating 1 cup of butter, 1/2 cup of powdered sugar, and a little vanilla until it gets smooth.
2. Now in a separate medium bowl, combine flour and the baking powder. Now add them to the butter mixture, then stir to mix, and then beat till well blended. Now stir in the pecans.
3. Into 1-inch balls, shape the dough and place it about 1 inch away on the buttered 12 x 15-inch sized baking sheets.
4. Now bake in 300º F convection oven till the cookies get pale golden brown, about 25 minutes. While baking two sheets at one time in one oven, then switch the positions halfway while baking. Let the cookies stand on the sheets until they are cool enough to be handled.
1. Lastly, place remaining of the 1 1/2 cups of powdered sugar in the shallow bowl. Then roll the warm cookies in the powdered sugar and coat all over them; discard the remaining sugar.
2. Place the cookies on racks to let them cool completely.

3. Serve.

## 6.11 Fresh Peach Pie Rock Creek Lake

Preparation time: 40 min | Servings: 8 | Difficulty: Medium

**Ingredients**

- Pastry
- Cream cheese, 1 package
- Sugar, 1 1/4 cups
- Firm-ripped peaches, 6 1/2 cups
- Orange juice, 3/4 cup
- Cornstarch, 1/4 cup
- Lemon juice, 1/4 cup

**Directions**

1. With the help of a fork, prick the bottom and also sides of the unbaked pastry in a pan 1-inch apart. Now bake in 375° convection oven till becomes golden, for about 15 to 20 minutes; now let cool on the rack.

2. Now, mix the cream cheese and 1/2 cup of sugar in a bowl until it gets smooth. Then spread it evenly over the bottom of the cool pastry.

3. In a food processor, now mix 1 cup of sliced peaches, the remaining 3/4 cup of sugar, some orange juice, and cornstarch until it gets smooth. Now pour into a 3 by 4-quart pan and stir in a medium-high heat till the mixture boils and also thickens, for about 4 minutes. Now remove from the heat and then stir in some lemon juice.

4. Now add the remaining 5 1/2 cups of peaches into the hot peach glaze and then mix and coat the slices. Now let them cool, for about 25 minutes, now scrape them onto the cream cheese mixture's crust.

5. Lastly, chill it uncovered, till it is firm enough to be cut, for 3 hours.

6. Cut into wedge-shape and then serve.

7. It can be inverted in a large bowl over the pie and be chilled up to almost 1 day.

## 6.12 Sweet and Hot Spiced Pecans

Preparation time: 45 | Servings: 8 | Difficulty: Medium

**Ingredients**

- Sugar, 1/3 cup
- Cayenne ,3/4 tsp
- Salt, 1/2 tsp
- Ground coriander, 1/2 tsp
- Ground cinnamon, 1/4 tsp
- Ground allspice, 1/8 tsp
- Egg white, 1 large
- Vegetable oil, 2 tbsp
- Pecan halves, 2 cups

**Directions**

1. Take a bowl and mix 1/3 cup of sugar, 3/4 tsp of cayenne, 1/2 tsp of Salt, 1/2 tsp of grounded coriander, 1/4 tsp of grounded cinnamon, and 1/8 tsp of grounded allspice. Now whisk in one egg white and two tbsp of vegetable oil. Now stir in two cups of pecan halves.

1. Now spread the nuts into a single layer in a nonstick oiled pan measuring 10- by 15-inch. Then bake in the 300° convection oven, keep on occasionally stirring, till the nuts become crisp and are lightly browned in color, 20 - 25 minutes.

2. Now let them cool for about 5 minutes, and then with a wide spatula, take the nuts out from the pan and cool them completely.

3. Lastly, serve or store them airtight at room temperature for up to almost two weeks.

## 6.13 Leek and Dubliner scones

Preparation time: 40 min | Servings: 5 | Difficulty: Medium

**Ingredients**

- Irish butter, 2 tbsps
- All-purpose flour, 2 1/4 cups
- Onion, 1 medium-sized
- Leek, 1 medium-sized
- Sugar, 1 tbsp
- Baking soda, 1/2 tsp
- Baking powder, 1/2 tsp
- Salt, 1/2 tsp
- Cold Irish butter, 1/4 cup
- Dubliner cheese, 1 cup
- Plain yogurt, 7 ounces

**Directions**

1. Start by preheating the oven to 390 °F in a convection oven. Now lightly oil and flour the baking sheet.
2. In a frying pan, melt the butter over medium heat, cook onion and leek, and keep on stirring until it gets soft and golden brown, for 5-7 minutes.
3. Now combine flour, baking soda, sugar, baking powder, salt in a food processor. Now add cheese, and then cut the butter till it looks like oatmeal. Now stir in onion and the leek mixture.
4. Keep some yogurt aside, mix some to make a dough, keeping it sticky but not very wet.

Now add some more yogurt if required.

5. Now transfer it to a work surface and then lightly knead it for a few seconds. Keep on patting it until it gets about 1-inch thick.
6. Lastly, cut out the 2-inch rounds and then place them on the cookie sheet.
7. Then transfer sheet to oven, bake it for 10-15 minutes.
8. Serve

## 6.14 Roasted Potato Rosemary Idaho with Apple Salad

Preparation time: 40 | Servings: 10 | Difficulty: Medium

**Ingredients**

- Idaho russet potatoes, 3 pounds
- Olive oil, 1/3 cup
- Fresh rosemary, 1/4 cup
- To taste Kosher salt.
- Black pepper fresh cracked
- Golden/Red apples, 4 each
- Lemon juice, 1/3 cup
- Dijon-style mustard, 1/4 cup
- Walnuts, 8 ounces

**Directions**

1. Place in a large bowl, potatoes, olive oil, salt, pepper, rosemary; place them in the sheet pan and then roast in 350°F temperature convection oven for 30-45 minutes or till it gets golden brown. Now remove from the heat and then let it cool. Cover it and chill.
2. Now wash, cut from the middle and dice the apples. Then combine with the potatoes in a large bowl.

3. Whisk together in the small bowl lemon juice, vinegar and also mustard till it gets smooth. Now pour it in the potato-apple mixture and then flip to coat them well. Now cover them and chill.

4. Stir in some walnuts and then mix well in a small bowl. Now adjust the seasonings with some salt and pepper.

5. Serve them as a composed salad or the platter salad as required.

## 6.15 Oat Bars Very Berry

Preparation time: 40 min | Servings: 40 bars | Difficulty: High

**Ingredients**

Cookie dough:

- Unsalted butter, 1 cup
- Granulated sugar, 1 cup
- Brown sugar packed, 1 cup.
- 2 eggs
- Pure vanilla extract, 1 tsp
- All-purpose flour, 1 cup
- Whole wheat flour, 1 cup
- Baking soda, 1 1/2 tsp
- Kosher salt, 1 tsp
- Ground cinnamon, 1 tsp
- Old-fashioned oats, 3 1/2 cups
- Raw quinoa, 1/4 cup
- Shredded unsweetened coconut, 1/2 cup

Berry mix-in:

- Frozen blackberries, 2 1/2 cups
- Honey, 3 tbsps
- Half of lemon zest
- Kosher salt, 1/4 tsp
- Ground black pepper

Berry glaze:

- Confectioner's sugar, 4 cups
- Pasteurized egg whites, 3
- Half of lemon zest
- Lemon juice, 2 tbsps
- Berry mix-in reserved

**Directions**

Cookie dough:

1. In a bowl with a stand mixer having a paddle attachment, mix the butter and some sugar. Now add cream and mix at a medium speed for almost 1 minute.
2. Now add egg, vanilla and cream and mix for 2 minutes on a medium-high.
3. Now add dry ingredients and then mix on low speed until it gets incorporated. However, do not overmix.
4. Now evenly spread almost 3/4 of the mixture in the half-sized sheet pan. Then distribute prepared berry mix in the cookie mix, now distribute remaining dough all over the fruit.
5. Then bake at the temperature of 325 °F in the convection oven for almost 20-25 min till the center is prepared. Cool bars completely, now leave them in the pan. Or you can cool them in the freezer.
6. After you cool them, then pour in the glaze over all the bars, spread with the offset spatula. Now allow frosting to set while keeping it uncovered.

7. Now cut into two by 2-inch squares and then serve.

Berry mix-in preparation:

1. Combine berries, pepper, honey, lemon in a small pot.
2. Then, cook in medium-low heat, stirring it occasionally, and smash the berries with spoon's back.
3. Now cook for almost 15 minutes or till the mixture gets thicken and berries have broken.
4. Now set them aside to cool, and reserve two tbsps.

Berry glaze preparation:

1. Combine egg whites, lemon juice, lemon zest, also remaining berry mix in the bowl containing a stand mixer with the whisk attachment.
2. Whisk for 30 seconds on medium speed.
3. Add the powdered sugar and beat on low until the sugar is just incorporated.
4. Now on medium speed beat for almost 2 minutes.
5. Glaze finished bars and serve.

## 6.16 Blossom Panna Cotta Yogurt-Orange

Preparation time: 40 | Servings: 1 | Difficulty: High

### Ingredients

The citrus salad

- Orange blossom honey, 3/4 cups
- Grapefruit juice, 1/3 cup
- Sweet wine, 2 tbsps
- Elderflower cordial, two tbsps
- Water, 1/4 cup
- Lime leaves, 3 kaffir

- Three limes, zest
- Pinch of salt
- Meyer lemon, grapefruit, tangerine segments and blood orange

The Sable Breton

- Butter, 3/4 cups
- Egg yolks, 4
- Sugar, 3/4 cups
- All-purpose flour, 1 cup
- Baking powder, 1 tbsp
- Salt, 1/2 tsp
- Beaten, 1 egg

The pistachio dragée

- Pistachios, 2/3 cups
- Confectioners' sugar, 1 tbsp
- Water, 1 tbsp
- Sugar, 1 1/2 tbsp
- Glucose, 1/4 tsp

For the Panna cotta

- Sugar, 4 tbsps
- Milk, 1/3 cup
- Gelatin, 4 sheets
- Vanilla yogurt, 2 1/4 cups
- 1 lime zest

- Orange blossom water, 1 tsp
- Citrus peels
- Vinegar
- Thyme leaves

**Directions**

The citrus salad

1. Start by heating the honey over medium heat in a small saucepan until it thickens and the color darkens, reducing to almost ¼ cup. Now deglaze with some grapefruit juice and some sweet wine.
2. Finally, add remaining ingredients except for segments, and then marinate overnight. Now strain it the next day; reheat to almost room temperature. Pour over them on the fresh segments.
3. Chill them before serving.

For the sable breton

1. Start by preheating the oven to almost 350 ° F.
2. Cream the butter in a bowl with an electric mixer is having paddle attachment on minimum speed until it is fluffy. Then, whisk attachment is fitted with a mixer and then put yolks and sugar in a separate bowl. Then whisk using low speed till pale and thick, then add to butter, and again beat together.
3. Now add the rest of the ingredients and mix, do not overmix. Now roll the dough till it is almost ¼-inch thick; cool it in the refrigerator. Now cut the discs to the same diameter, i.e., 4-ounce ramekin.
4. Now brush it with egg wash, transfer to oven, and then bake until it gets golden brown, 10-20 minutes in the conventional oven.
5. Re-trim them when still warm and then let cool.

The pistachio dragée

1. Start by preheating the oven to almost 275 °F.
2. Now lightly toast pistachios in the oven for almost 5 minutes; do not brown. Now toss in the bowl with some confectioners' sugar; set it aside. Now heat the water, glucose and sugar in the saucepan at 285 °F measured by a candy thermometer. Now add the nuts; stir them to coat.
3. Pour onto the Silpat and then immediately remove them to the bowl.

The panna cotta

1. In the saucepan, heat sugar and milk at medium heat till it becomes hot. Now soak gelatin in ice water for almost 10 minutes, and then squeeze the excess water out and then add the hot milk. Now remove it from the heat and then allow the milk to cool at room temperature.
2. Now stir the vanilla yogurt, orange blossom, lime zest, and water and then pour into the ramekin/mold. Allow setting in the refrigerator.
3. Once it is set, then carefully unmold in the serving bowl. Invert and release one edge.
4. Now place panna cotta on the top of sable Breton. Arrange citrus salad with it. Then sprinkle pistachio dragée on the top and then garnish it with some citrus peels, thyme leaves and balsamic vinegar.

## 6.17 Quinoa Sticky Toffee Pudding

Preparation time: 40 | Servings: 6 | Difficulty: High

### Ingredients

For the cake:

- Dates pitted, 9 ounces.
- Water, 1 ½ cup
- Cinnamon sticks, 3 whole
- All-purpose flour, 6 ounces
- Toasted quinoa flour, 4 ounces

- Salt, ¾ tsp
- Butter, 3 ounces
- Sugar, 5 ounces
- 3 eggs
- Vanilla extract, 1 ½ tsp
- Baking soda, 1 ½ tsp
- For the sauce:
- Dark brown sugar, 1 ½ cup
- Molasses, 6 tbsps
- Honey, 6 tbsps
- Butter, ¾ pound
- Heavy cream ¾ cup

**Directions**

Cake

1. Start by preheating the oven to almost 325 ° F.
2. Now bring some dates, cinnamon sticks and water to boil and then simmer until dates are broken down a little for about 5 minutes.
3. Mix the flour, salt and quinoa flour in a separate bowl.
4. Now cream butter and sugar till it is light and fluffy, now add in eggs and the vanilla. Do it in the standing mixer with a paddle attachment.
5. Now remove cinnamon from the date mixture and purée it until it gets smooth. Then put it in the bowl and then mix in with the baking soda; and set aside.
6. Now add the remaining dry mixture with date mixture, and then mix it until it is combined.
7. Now pour the batter in a well-sprayed pan and then bake till set, for about 20 - 25 minutes

in the convection oven.

Sauce:

1. Add and combine all of the ingredients, bring them to boil. Now reduce the heat and then let it simmer for almost 2 to 3 minutes.

2. After the cake is baked, cool it slightly and cut it to the pan's desired size. Now poke holes in the top of the cake and then cover it completely with prepared sauce. Let it sit for almost 30 minutes and soak in the sauce

3. Serve.

## 6.18 Sour Cream Cardamom Cake

Preparation time: 40 | Servings: 6 | Difficulty: High

**Ingredients**

- Terra-cotta pot, 1 unglazed
- Cooking parchment, 1 piece
- Butter, ¾ cup
- Sugar, 1 ¼ cups
- Eggs, 3 larges
- Sour cream, 1 cup
- All-purpose flour, 2 ½ cups
- Golden raisins, 1 cup
- Baking powder, 1 ½ tbsp
- Baking soda, ½ tsp
- Ground cardamom, ½ tsp
- Sliced almonds, 3 tbsps

**Directions**

1. Start by washing the pot with the soap and water and then dry well. Now line the pot with the cooking parchment by pushing the center of the parchment into the pot, press it outward to fit the pot's contours, and bend the parchment edges outward over the edges of the pot.

2. Beat the butter and sugar in a bowl with a mixer until it gets fluffy. Now add eggs and then beat it until it is well blended. Now turn the mixer to a medium and beat in the sour cream.

3. Mix the flour, baking powder, raisins, baking soda, and the cardamom in another bowl. Now add to the butter mixture and then beat them on medium speed until it gets well blended. Now scrape the batter into the parchment-lined with the pot. Then sprinkle on the almonds very evenly.

4. Now set the cake in the lower third level of the 300° convection oven. Place it on an inverted baking pan, lift the cake slightly so the bottom is not brown. If the parchment touches the top of the oven, fold it down farther over the pot edges. Then bake it until it is a long wooden skewer inserted in the center of the cake that comes out clean, for about 1 1/2 to almost 1 3/4 hours.

5. Now cool the cake in the pot on the rack for almost 15 - 20 minutes, lift it from the pot and then set upright. Now cool it at least for 1 1/2 hours longer. Return the cake to the pot for presentation.

6. Lift the cake from the pot, peel off the parchment, and then cut into wedges.

7. Serve.

# Chapter 7: Turkey

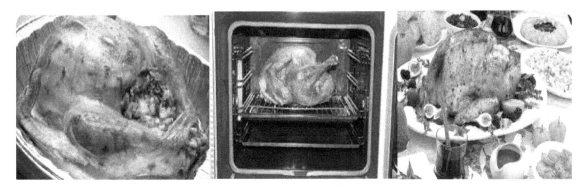

## 7. 1 Turkey Picnic Loaf Jerk-spiced

Preparation time: 1 hr. 50 min | Servings: 8 | Difficulty: Medium

**Ingredients**

- Mushrooms, 8 ounces
- Onion, 1
- Salad oil, 2 tbsps
- Salt, 1/2 tsp
- Ground nutmeg, 1/2 tsp
- Ground allspice ,1/2 tsp
- Ground cinnamon 1/4 tsp
- Cayenne, 1/4 tsp
- Cider, 3 tbsps
- Molasses, 2 tbsps
- All-purpose flour, 1/2 cup
- Ground turkey, 1 1/2 pounds

- Chicken broth, 1/2 cup
- Egg, 1 large
- Drained onions, 3/4 cup
- Paper-thin prosciutto about 6 ounces

**Directions**

1. In a 10 by 12-inch pan over high heat, stir the mushrooms and some onion in two tbsps oil till begins to brown, for 7 - 8 minutes.
2. Now add salt, cinnamon, nutmeg, allspice, and cayenne; then stir until it is fragrant, 2 minutes. Now add vinegar and also molasses, then stir often till the liquid is evaporated completely. Then scrape into the large bowl, add flour, and mix it to blend, often stir till it is lukewarm, almost 5 minutes.
3. Add the turkey, egg, broth to the bowl, then mix well. Now gently stir it in pickled onions.
4. Now oil the 5 x 9-inch nonstick pan. Line the pan neatly with the single layer of the prosciutto slices, now overlap the edges slightly, and then press the prosciutto's ends against the pan sides, but not over the rim. Now scrape the meat mixture into the pan and then gently pat to level. Then fold the ends of the prosciutto slices neatly all oven meat.
5. Now bake the turkey loaf in 350° convection oven till the thermometer inserted in the center of the thickest part reaches almost 160°, and the meat is no longer pinky in the shade, almost 55 minutes; then loaf will begin shrinking from the pan sides.
6. Lastly, Let stand it at room temperature for at least 10 minutes. Then Invert it in a slightly larger, rimmed platter over the pan; then hold the pan and the platter together and now invert. Lastly, lift the pan to release the loaf.

## 7.2. Classic Roast Turkey

Preparation time: 1 hr. 50 min | Servings: 8 | Difficulty: Medium

**Ingredients**

- 1 turkey
- Melted butter
- Olive oil classic gravy

**Directions**

1. First, remove and discard the leg truss from the turkey. Now pull off and then discard any of the lumps of fat. Then remove the giblets and neck and save them for classic gravy. Then rinse the turkey, and pat dry. Now rub the turkey with butter.

2. Now place the turkey keeping the breast up, in a V-shaped rack of 12 x17-inch roasting pan. Insert meat thermometer through the straight down the thickest part of the breast to bone.

3. Now roast in a convection oven until the thermometer registers at almost 160° C.

4. If the turkey is unstuffed, then tip it slightly to drain all juices from the body cavity into the pan. Transfer the turkey to the platter. Let them stand in a warm place, keep it uncovered for almost 20 to 30 minutes, and then carve it. If the thigh joints are pink, then cut the drumsticks from the thighs and place thighs in the baking pan, bake at 450° oven till it is no longer pink, for 10 - 15 minutes, or you can put on a microwave-safe plate, cook in the microwave oven at the full power for about 1 to 3 minutes.

5. Serve with Classic Gravy.

## 7.3. Thanksgiving Mayonnaise Roasted Turkey

Preparation time: 3 hr. 15 min | Servings: 14 | Difficulty: Medium

**Ingredients**

- 1 turkey
- Oregano, 6 stems
- Pepper freshly ground
- Salt
- Rosemary, 6 stems
- Leaves, 14 sage
- Celery, 6 stalks
- Onions, 2 large
- Mayonnaise, 1 1/2 jars
- Fresh thyme, 12 stems
- Salted butter, 1 stick

**Directions**

1. Preheat up to 450° F in oven. Be sure that the turkey is thawed; you need to cut all the bad parts inside that are bundled in. Rinse it inside and out deeply, and then pats it fully dry. Now scatter about the third part of the sliced celery and onions at the roasting pan's bottom.

2. Strip the leaves from all the stems and cut thinly, and blend properly with mayonnaise. Prepare yourself to get sloppy. Turn the turkey over and work there on the bottom, spreading the mixture of mayonnaise and herbs across the skin but in all crevices. You have to salt that surface and spice it then liberally. Flip, inside of the bird, do the same. Generously season.

3. Stuff a third of celery and onions and then a stick of the butter with the bird. Scatter the

remainder on top, bring it in the oven, and roast for half an hour at 450 °F. Turn the oven down to 350 ° F and then cook for two and a half hours.

## 7.4. Rosemary and thyme flavored turkey

Preparation time: 3 hr. 15 min | Servings: 12 | Difficulty: Easy

**Ingredients**

- 1 whole turkey
- Vegetable oil, 1/2 cup
- Fresh rosemary
- Fresh thyme

**Directions**

1. Start by preheating the oven to almost 350 ° F on a convection setting.
2. Then wash turkey from inside and out and then pat dry it with paper towels.
3. Now Place the turkey on the roasting pan and then brush it with olive oil.
4. Then Cut and also loosen skin from the turkey breast and then rub it with rosemary and also thyme over the turkey.
5. Lastly, Place turkey in the lowest rack of the oven and then cook for almost 2-2 1/2 hours until turkey thighs' internal temperature reaches almost 180 ° F.
6. Serve.

## 7.5. Spatchcocked Turkey served with Herb Butter and Flavored Gravy

Preparation Time: 2h 5m | Serves: 8 | Difficulty: Easy

**Ingredients**

- Onions, peeled and chopped, 4 larges
- Carrots, peeled and chopped, 4 larges

- Celery, roughly chopped, 6 stalks
- Thyme sprigs, 12
- Turkey, 1 whole
- Herb butter, 1/2 c
- Vegetable oil, 2 tbsp.
- Kosher salt and black pepper
- Chicken broth, 1 1/2 qt
- Bay leaves, 2
- . Butter, 3 tbsp
- Flour, 4 tbsp.
- Herb Butter
- Chopped sage, 1 tbsp.
- Chopped thyme, 1 tbsp.
- Traeger poultry rub, 1 tbsp
- Softened butter, 1/2 c

**Directions**

1. Adjust the oven rack's center location and preheat the oven to 450 ° F. Use an aluminum foil to cover the rimmed baking sheet or the broiler plate. Scatter the bottom of the plate with two-thirds of the cabbage, broccoli, celery & thyme sprigs. Directly place the slotted broiler rack/ wire rack on the top of the vegetables.

2. Dry the turkey with the paper towels and brush with butter on both surfaces. Season it liberally with salt and black pepper across all surfaces (dismiss salting phase if brined, salted, or the Kosher turkey is used). Tuck tips of the wing behind the back. Position the turkey on the top of a rack, positioning so that the sides may not overlap, pulling back on the breastbone to flatten the breasts gently.

3. Move the turkey to oven and then cook, spin it occasionally for around 80 minutes unless an instant-read thermometer placed in the deepest part of breast registers almost150 ° F and the thighs register at around 165 ° F.

4. Create the stuffing while the turkey roasts. Slice the spine, backbone, and giblets loosely. Heat the remaining 1 tbsp of oil in a 3-quart saucepan until it shimmers, of er high heat. Attach the diced turkey pieces and simmer for around 5 minutes, stirring regularly, until lightly browned. Attach the remaining onions, carrots and celery and proceed to cook for another 5 minutes, stirring regularly, before the vegetables begin to soften and brown in places. Add the stock of chicken, left thyme, and the bay leaves. Carry to the boil, bring to a mere simmer and reduce. Enable 45 minutes to cook, then strain into the 2-quart fluid measuring cup via a fine-mesh strainer and discard solids. Skim off some fat from the broth's crust.

5. Melt butter in a 2-quart saucepan over medium-high flame. Connect the flour and cook for around 3 minutes, stirring continuously until the flour is golden brown. Add broth in a small, continuous stream until everything has incorporated, whisking constantly. Bring to the boil, reduce it to simmer, and then cook for around 20 minutes longer until lowered to about 1 cup. Season with salt and pepper to taste, cover, and keep it warm with the gravy.

6. Remove the turkey from the oven and switch the rack to a fresh baking sheet when the turkey is baked. Give 20 minutes to rest before carving at room temperature. In a liquid measuring cup, gently squeeze any gathered juices from the roasting pan thru the fine-mesh strainer. Skim and discard extra fat. Whisk the gravy juices down.

# Chapter 8: Fish

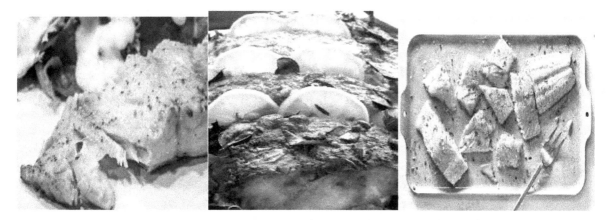

## 8.1 Fish Tacos

Preparation Time: 2h 5m | Serves: 8 | Difficulty: Easy

**Ingredients**

- Napa Cabbage, 3 Cups
- Kraft Mayo, 1/4 C, with Olive Oil
- lime juice 2 tbsp
- Breaded fish filets oven-ready, 1 package
- Corn tortillas, 12
- Salt and pepper as needed

**Directions**

1. First, cook the fish according to the package directions. Now stir it together with cabbage, and lime juice and mayo; set aside.

2. Now wrap the tortillas in the aluminum foil and then warm in the oven during the last 10 minutes of the fish cooking time. Now remove the fish from the oven and then cut each of the filets into six chunks.

3. Lastly, Place three pieces of the fish on each tortilla, then top it with almost two tbsps of the cabbage mixture. Then Serve with the Baja Sauce, some salsa, or the guacamole. It will Serve 6.

## 8.2. Grilled Garlic Salmon

Preparation Time: 35m | Serves: 5 | Difficulty: Easy

**Ingredients**

- Salmon fillet, one large cut to the pan size
- Garlic3 cloves (or to taste)
- Lemon pepper, 1/2-1 tbsp.
- Garlic salt, 1/2 tbsp.
- Butter, 1 tbsp
- Olive oil, 2 tbsp
- Milk, 1/2 cup

**Directions**

1. First, rinse the fillet with 1/2 C of milk. If the fish has a stronger odor (or you do not like the fishy taste), you can set in the milk for almost up to 5 minutes. Then Preheat the oven to almost 350 ° F.

2. In the oven-proof skillet, start by melting butter and the oil until hot. Now add in the garlic, i.e., finely minced. Now place in the fish, with skin side down, brown it for 1 minute. Now dust the flesh side of the fish with the garlic salt and some lemon pepper. Then Flip and also brown for about 1 minute. Now place the fish skin down in the pan, transfer the entire pan to the oven pre-heated at almost 350 ° F. Now roast for about 5 min per inch of the fillet thickness in medium fish, almost 10 min per inch for the well-done fish.

3. Serve and Enjoy.

## 8.3 Fish Parsley Pesto

Preparation Time: 17 min | Serves: 4 | Difficulty: Easy

**Ingredients**

Pesto:

- Flat-leaf parsley, one bunch, leaves only, chopped
- Minced, 1 garlic clove
- Olive oil, 2 tbsp
- Zested and juiced, 1 lemon,
- Whole-wheat breadcrumbs 2 tbsps
- Black pepper, 1/2 tsp
- White-fleshed fish fillet, 16 ounces, 6-8 ounces each, 2 fillets approx.

**Directions**

Pesto:

1. First, place parsley in the small food processor, then pulse 6-8 times. Then Add the remaining constituents, then process till it gets thick in the sauce forms. (Keep the Sauce in a sealed container for almost up to 1 week.)

Fish:

2. To 400 °F, pre-heat the oven. Over the high fire, put the cast iron skillet. With paper towels, wipe the fish off. Spritz the fish gently with nonstick cooking spray on all sides. Transfer the fish to a pan until the skillet is heated. For 2-3 minutes per side, fry. Cover each fish partly with 1/4 of the cup of pesto. To steam the sauce, move that pan to an oven for five min. Note that within the oven, your pan's handle can get heated!

3. Allows 1 cup of sauce, 1/4 cup each serving: Three ounces of fried fish each serving, roughly.

## 8.4 Homemade Fish Sticks

Preparation Time: 20 min | Serves: 4 | Difficulty: Easy

**Ingredients**

- Fish fillets, 1 pound
- 1 egg
- Breadcrumbs, 1/3 cup
- Grated parmesan cheese, 1/3 cup
- Dried parsley, 1/2 tbsp
- Paprika, 1/2 tbsp
- Melted, 1 tbsp butter

**Directions**

1. Pre-heat the oven to 450 ° C.
2. Beat the egg in a shallow bowl. Place some breadcrumbs, grated parmesan, paprika & parsley in another shallow bowl.
3. Slice the fish (approximately 3 inches long and 1/2 inches wide) between strips.
4. Into egg, plunge each strip, and then onto the crumb mix.
5. Place the strips of fish on a baking sheet that is lightly greased.
6. Drizzle over the fish with the molten butter.
7. Now, Bake it with the fork for about 7-10 minutes or till the fish flakes rapidly.

## 8.5 Baked Parmesan Swai

Preparation Time: 20 m | Serves: 2 | Difficulty: Easy

**Ingredients**

- Swai Filet, 12 oz

- Oil, 2 Tbsp
- fresh Thyme, 1 tsp
- Rosemary, 1 tsp
- Lemon Juice approx. an oz
- grated Parmesan Cheese, 2 tbsps

**Directions**

1. Pre-heat the oven to 350° F.
2. In a glass baking dish, add olive oil into the base.
3. Now sprinkle thyme and Rosemary into Oil
4. When the fish is thawed, lie down in the baking dish and then turn over.
5. Sprinkle over the tuna with lemon juice
6. Parmesan cheese in the dust over fish
7. Bake for fifteen minutes,
8. Whenever it's transparent and flakes quickly with a fork, the fish would be cooked.

## 8.6 Garlic Roasted Mahi Mahi

Preparation Time: 23 m | Serves: 1 | Difficulty: Easy

**Ingredients**

- Mahi Mahi, 2-4 pieces
- Garlic Olive Oil, 1/2-1 tbsp
- Dill
- Roasted Garlic

**Directions**

1. Start by pre-heating the oven to 350 ° F.

2. Now take 2-4 pieces of the filleted Mahi Mahi. Then Make tiny slits on top of every piece of the fish. Now pour the 1/2-1 tbsp of the garlic flavor olive oil all over fish, then sprinkle with the roasted garlic and some dill (the amount used for roasted Garlic and dill can change depending on the taste required).

3. Now, place the fish in oven to Bake for almost 15-20 minutes.

## 8.7 Geraine's Mahi Mahi Ginger Soy

Preparation Time: 40 m | Serves: 4 | Difficulty: Easy

**Ingredients**

- Brown sugar, 3 tbsps
- Water, 4 tbsp
- Soy sauce, 2 tbsps
- Balsamic vinegar, 1 tbsp
- Ground ginger, 2 tbsp
- Minced garlic, 1 tsp
- Olive oil, 1 tsp
- Mahi mahi fillets, 1 1/4 lb. cut in 4
- Salt, pepper to taste

**Directions**

1. Stir the sugar, some balsamic vinegar, water, some soy sauce, ginger and garlic and the olive oil with each other in a small glass container.

2. Mildly season your fish fillets with some salt and pepper, and then put them in the dish.

3. Cover them, then refrigerate them to marinate for about 20 minutes (having turned after 10 minutes).

4. Now, Preheat the oven to almost 350 F.

5. Now, Take the fish from the tray. Pour the retained marinade into the pan when the fish is baking and then decrease until the mixture falls into the glaze. Now Leave it aside to set.

6. Now, put the fish on the baking tray and then bake it for almost 10 minutes till the fish flakes. Spread fillets on the serving dish with the spoonful of the glaze over fish and then serve warm. Incorporate some wild rice and some colorful vegetable and also salad.

7. Enjoy

# Chapter 9: Pizza

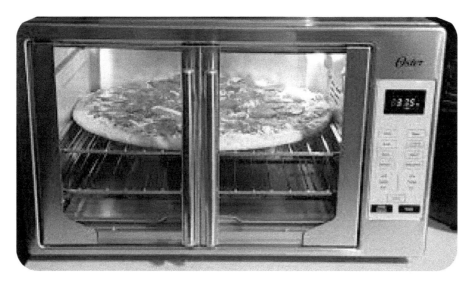

## 9.1 Cheese Pizza Recipe

Preparation Time: 60 min | Servings: 6 | Difficulty: Medium

**Ingredients**

- Pizza base 2, readymade
- Tomato ketchup, 1 1/2 tbsp
- Black pepper, 1 pinch, ground
- Mozzarella, 150 gm, shredded
- Salt, 1/2 tsp

For Toppings

- Onion 100 gm, sliced
- Capsicum 70 gm, sliced
- Tomato 100 gm, sliced
- Mushroom 50 gm, sliced

**Directions**

1. Pre-heat the oven in convection mode at about 250 º F to prepare this wonderful cheese pizza recipe. In the meanwhile, distribute the tomato sauce uniformly per each pizza base. Now take the chopping board and cut the carrots, the peppers, the capsicum and the mushroom.

2. Microwave the vegetables for about one minute.

3. In a pan, mix all the sliced vegetables with the seasoning. Now microwave all these vegetables for about 30-40 seconds or maybe one minute in a dish which is a microwave-safe dish. Spread the vegetable topping on the base of each pizza. Spray the finely chopped mozzarella cheese on top of each slice.

4. Bake the pizza for around 10-12 minutes.

5. You can use the microwave for baking this pizza, or you can also use the nonstick Tawa. Nevertheless, we used the microwave in our recipe. Bake your pizza on the top rack at 250 º F before the cheese is melted. It's going to take about 10-12 mins. Slice the yummy Cheese Pie into pieces and then serve with sauces. Enjoy

## 9.2 Vegetable pizza

Preparation Time: 30 min | Servings: 4 | Difficulty: Easy

**Ingredients**

- For making Pizza Dough
  - Dry Yeast, 1 tsp
  - Water Warm, 1/4 Cup
  - All-Purpose Flour or Maida, 160 g
  - White Salt, 1/2 tsp
  - Olive Oil, 3/2 tbsp

For Pizza Topping

- Sweet Tomato Sauce 1 tbsp, you can also use Pizza Sauce
- Tomato 1, 3-inch diameter, round shaped
- Green Bell Pepper Capsicum 1, 3.5-inch diameter, round shaped
- Mozzarella Cheese, 100 g
- Olive Oil, 1 tbsp
- White Salt, 1/4 tsp

**Directions**

1. Dip the yeast in about 30 ml of hot water. Shake well to make it dissolve properly with water. Now sift the Maida in a wide tub. Add the salt, the oil and then the yeast mixture into the flour. To make a soft dough, we have to add water and then knead it continuously slowly. It'll take around 4-5 minutes to knead; then, a nice smooth dough will be ready.
2. Take another bowl and add half a tbsp of oil to grease. Add the dough now.
3. Roll this over once to make certain that this dough ball is fully coated with greased oil.
4. Close the top of the container and ferment for about 1 hour at room temperature.
5. After one hour, produce a medium-size pizza about 9 inches in diameter with a half-inch width.
6. Add 1/2 tbsp of oil to the baking sheet and grease thoroughly.
7. Put this pizza cautiously in a greased baking dish.
8. Label Minor cuts on the top of the pizza by using a knife. Now it will allow the cheese to get melt and hit the interior of Pizza bread.
9. Pre-heat now the microwave convection for the baking purpose
10. Once we start decorating our pizza, just do some other multi-tasking, so to save

our time, we will pre-heat the microwave.

11. Pre-heating is an essential aspect of the cooking process. Usually, it's required to get the microwave to the predefined temperature right before placing something to bake. It allows us to achieve optimum results and bake the bread at the correct temperature during cooking.

12. We like to pre-heat this at 392 ° F.

13. Put the vegetables & chicken and then cover it all with the cheese.

14. Cast the tomato sauce all over the pizza crust, excluding corners with the aid of a spoon.

15. Dispersed the sauce around the pizza surface.

16. Now, put the rings of tomatoes, the capsicum and the baby corn. Sprinkle with a little pinch of salt or as required over the pizza.

17. Sprinkle the whole pizza with the cheese.

18. Pour 1/2 tsp of oil over the top of your pizza. It is not approved for a weak heart or nutrition-conscious mega models. If you like, you can bypass this phase.

Baking Pizza using Microwave Convection oven.

1. It will take 20 minutes for baking pizza.

2. Set the oven to 392 ° F pre-heat level. Put on the Microwave safety gloves and then dig in the pizza inside the pre-heated microwave.

Baking pizza in Convection mode of microwave

3. Close the microwave/oven door and baked at 392 ° F for 20 minutes.

4. After 20 minutes, turn off your Microwave / Oven, then pull out the pizza. Make sure to keep your gloves dry. The delicious hot pizza is about to be eaten. Enjoy!

## 9.3 Chicken cheese pizza

Preparation Time: 1 hour 40 min | Servings: 4-6 | Difficulty: Medium

**Ingredients**

For making Pizza Dough

- Dry Yeast, 1 tsp
- Water Warm, 1/4 Cup
- Fried chicken 1/2 cup, cut into pieces
- All Purpose flour or maida, 160 g
- White Salt, 1/2 tsp
- Olive Oil, 3/2 tbsp Oil

For Pizza Topping

- Sweet Tomato Sauce 1 tbsp, you can also use Pizza Sauce
- Tomato 1, 3-inch diameter, Round shaped
- Green Bell Pepper Capsicum 1, 3.5-inch diameter, round shaped
- Mozzarella Cheese, 100 g
- Olive Oil, 1 tbsp
- White Salt, 1/4 tsp
- Red Chili Flakes, 1 tsp
- Baby Corn Sticks 4, Each corn cut into 2 pieces from the center; it's optional

**Directions**

1. Dip the yeast in about 30 ml of hot water. Shake well to make it dissolve properly with water. Now sift the Maida in a wide tub. Add the salt, the oil and then the yeast mixture into the flour. To make a soft dough, we have to add water and then knead it continuously slowly. It'll take around 4-5 minutes to knead; then, a nice

smooth dough will be ready.

2. Take another bowl and add half a tbsp of oil to grease. Add the dough now.

3. Roll this over once to make certain that this dough ball is fully coated with greased oil.

4. Close the top of the container and ferment for about 1 hour at room temperature.

5. After one hour, produce a medium-size pizza about 9 inches in diameter with a half-inch width.

6. Add 1/2 tbsp of oil to the baking sheet and grease thoroughly.

7. Put this pizza cautiously in a greased baking dish.

8. Label Minor cuts on the top of the pizza by using a knife. Now it will allow the cheese to get melt and hit the interior of Pizza bread.

9. Pre-heat now the microwave convection for the baking purpose

10. Once we start decorating our pizza, just do some other multi-tasking, so to save our time, we will pre-heat the microwave.

11. Pre-heating is an essential aspect of the cooking process. Usually, it's required to get the microwave to the predefined temperature right before placing something to bake. It allows us to achieve optimum results and bake the bread at the correct temperature during cooking.

12. We like to pre-heat this at 392 ° F.

13. Put the vegetables & chicken and then cover it all with the cheese.

14. Cast the tomato sauce all over the pizza crust, excluding corners with the aid of a spoon.

15. Dispersed the sauce around the pizza surface.

16. Now, put the rings of tomatoes, the capsicum and the baby corn. Sprinkle with a little pinch of salt or as required over the pizza.

17. Sprinkle the whole pizza with the cheese.

18. Pour 1/2 tsp of oil over the top of your pizza. It is not approved for a weak heart or nutrition-conscious mega models. If you like, you can bypass this phase.

Baking Pizza using Microwave Convection oven.

1. It will take 20 minutes for baking pizza.

2. At this point, you're Microwave / Oven was supposed to hit the 392 °F pre-heat level. Put on the Microwave safety gloves and then dig in the pizza inside a pre-heated microwave.

3. Closed the microwave/oven door and baked at a temperature of 392 °F for 20 minutes.

4. After 20 minutes, turn off your Microwave / Oven, then pull out the pizza. Make sure to keep your gloves dry. The delicious hot pizza is about to be eaten. Enjoy.

# Chapter 10: Snacks

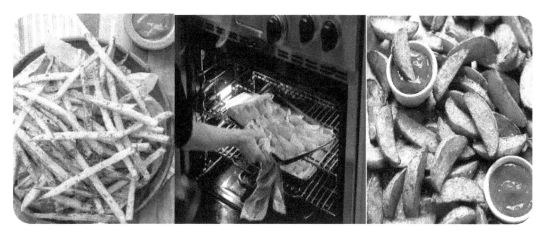

## 10.1. Oven fries

Preparation Time: 40 min | Servings: 4 | Difficulty: Easy

**Ingredients**

- Baking potatoes, 4 medium
- Cooking spray
- Olive oil, 1 tbsp
- Salt, 1 tsp

**Directions**

1. Start by preheating the oven to 425 °F in a convection oven.
2. Now Peel potatoes and then slice them into strips.
3. Generously coat the baking sheet with the cooking spray. Now arrange the potato strips in a single layer in the baking tray.
4. Now drizzle the potatoes with some olive oil and then sprinkle some salt. Now bake for almost 30 minutes, or until it gets golden brown and becomes crunchy.

## 10.2. Roasted potatoes

Preparation Time: 35 min | Servings: 6 | Difficulty: Easy

**Ingredients**

- Potatoes 2 pounds, i.e., 1 kg, might be Russet, Red or Yukon Gold.
- Vegetable oil, 2 tbsps
- Salt, 1/4 tsp
- Black pepper, 1/2 tsp should be freshly ground.
- Thyme, 1 tsp should be fresh and finely chopped.
- Rosemary, 1 tsp should be fresh and finely chopped.
- Fleur de sel, you might take fine salt (a pinch), Optional.
- Rosemary and thyme with herb blossoms

Sour cream dip:

- Sour cream about 1/2 cup, as per choice you can take more
- Parsley 2 tbsp, should be fresh and finely chopped
- Salt & black pepper, as per taste
- Chili flakes for heating, Optional

**Directions**

1. Thoroughly wash and clean the potatoes well. Cut the potatoes into about 3/4 to 1-inch cubes. Note that potatoes should be reasonably cut for frying.
2. Put oil, salt, pepper, thyme and rosemary in a big cup. Whisk with a fork before it's well mixed.
3. Transfer the potatoes into the mixing bowl and mix well till they are finely coated. Line 2 baking sheets of parchment paper. Place the potatoes over the lined baking sheets. Ensure the potatoes are well laid out or don't blend or cook unevenly and even do not become crispy.

4. Bake the potatoes in a hot oven of 390 ° F (200 ° C) fan or a convection oven. Use 425 ° F when using an oven having top and bottom heating components. Bake for about 15 minutes, then cut the sheets and rotate the potatoes. Now again, bake for 5-10 minutes or till the potatoes become crispy, lightly browned and cooked through, based on the size. Keep in mind that potatoes become brown uniformly from all sides in convection ovens, but it might not be the same for an oven having top and bottom heating components. Rotate the sheets in half.

5. Serve right away while it is still hot. Complete the baked potatoes recipe with fleur de sel and perhaps a pinch of standard fine salt, based on your palate. End up serving with either a dip of sour cream or with your dip sauce.

For the dip of the sour cream:

1. Add all of the ingredients to the mixing bowl and stir well.

2. In case you have leftovers: the baked potatoes taste fantastic in comparison to salads or cups.

## 10.3. Simple Bacon

Preparation Time: 23 min | Servings: 2 | Difficulty: Easy

**Ingredients**

- Bacon, 8-10 slices
- Aluminum foil, for covering tray
- Parchment paper, in case, needed

**Directions**

1. Preheat the oven to the convection of 400 °F or 425 °F. You may begin with the cold oven and, in this case, add a couple of minutes. If you like, you may use a slightly high or even low oven temperature, which will take some more or fewer minutes, depending on the case.

2. Take an 18 × 13-inch studded sheet pan and line it with a wide aluminum foil sheet; prefer heavy-duty foil. Put the bacon over the sheet next to each other but still not touching each other. Up to 9-10 bits, around 1/2 pounds, normally suit. If you have trouble sticking or utilizing thinner bacon, in that case, parchment paper might be a safer option.

3. Place it in the center of the oven. You can do something else for the next 18 minutes, then come here. Time can differ depending on how thick the bacon is, the temperature of your oven and your taste. Now it's done if it looks done.

4. Discharge on paper towels, then pat "dry" using another paper towel.

## 10.4. Popovers

Preparation Time: 50 min | Servings: 2-3 | Difficulty: medium

**Ingredients**

- Eggs, 3
- Milk, 1 cup
- Canola Oil, 3 tbsp
- All-purpose flour, 1 cup
- Kosher salt, 1/2 tsp.
- Popover Pan

**Directions**

1. Preheat the oven for about 400 °F in either the convection or the baking mode, or only roast.

2. Spray the cooking spray (should be non-stick one) on the popover pan before preparing the batter, then put this pan in the oven and heat it.

3. In case the eggs and the milk are not placed at room temperature, then heat the eggs after removing from shells for around 12 to15 sec. and the milk for around 20-30 sec. in the

microwave oven

4. Whisk together the chicken and milk with oil. Combine flour, then add it to the mixture of eggs. Add the salt, then blend the mixture till it becomes smooth and clear of any clumps.
5. Remove the popover pan from the oven, then put a little butter inside each of the popover cups.
6. For every popover cup, pour the batter almost 3/4 full way. If you run low and one cup among all is empty, then add water filling up of about 1/2 way.
7. Now put this filled pan inside the oven of 400 ° F, then bake for 20 minutes in case of convection oven baking and for conventional bake, bake it for about 30 minutes, after cooking for about 20 to 30 minutes.
8. Then, after the oven door is locked, turn down the oven's heat to 325 ° F.
9. At this moment, if you are cooking on the convection mode, then turn to bake mode. Cook for another five to 15 minutes by keeping an eye on the popovers.
10. You are going to realize that they are finished when they transform into a pretty golden brown.
11. Serve right away.

## 10.5. Convection Oven Granola

Preparation Time: 55 min | Servings: 5 | Difficulty: Easy

**Ingredients**

- Rolled oats, 1 1/2 cups
- Slivered almonds or whole if you like 1/2 cup
- Pecans, 1/2 cup
- Walnuts 1/4 cup optional -- use 1/4 cup oats extra in case you don't have walnuts

- Toasted wheat germ, 2 tbsp if you have it
- Salt, 3/8 tsp
- Egg white medium 1, lightly beaten by a fork
- Light brown sugar, 3 scant tbsps
- Maple syrup, 2 tbsps
- Honey, 1 tbsp
- Walnut oil, 2 tbsps, coconut oil, may also be used
- Vanilla, 1/2 tsp

**Directions**

1. Start with preheating the convection oven to a temperature of about 275 º F. Then, line a large, high and rimmed cookie sheet with the parchment paper.

2. In a large mixing bowl, combine the wheat germ, almonds, walnuts, pecans, and the rolled oats. Simply add salt, then stir to disperse the salt evenly.

3. Add the egg white into the oat mixture, then stir it well.

4. Inside a microwave-safe measuring cup, combine brown sugar, maple syrup, honey and the oil. Heat on high flame for about 1 minute; after this, stir to diffuse the sugar slightly. Stir the vanilla. Pour the hot syrup blend over the granola, then stir it till the mixture is evenly coated. Drain the oat mixture over the two cookie sheets, now spread it as uniformly as possible, then press down marginally in a way that the oats are in the finely thin and tightly packed layer.

5. Now, bake it in the convection oven for about 35 to 45 mins, preventing mixing every 15 minutes. Note that the granola must be nicely golden brown, whereas it's still somewhat soft once you remove it from the oven. It's supposed to crisp up when it cools.

## 10.6. Roasted vegetables

Preparation Time: 35 min | Servings: 5-6 | Difficulty: Medium

**Ingredients**

- Vegetables of choice, 1-2 lbs.
- Terra delyssa / olive oil, 1 - 2 tbsps
- Sea salt and black pepper with some other spices as per taste

**Directions**

1. Preheat your oven to a temperature of 425 ° F. Let the oven preheat fully. Arrange the rack at the center location.
2. Wash and completely dry the vegetables properly (dried vegetables can roast much smoother, so hold them in check). Peel, cut and slice into reasonably standard bits if needed.
3. Draw the vegetables onto the baking sheet on a single line so as not to clutter the pot. Plenty of vegetables won't roast but will finish steaming.
4. Rub the olive oil (or any oil of your choice) on the vegetables or spray them and mix well to cover uniformly.
5. Season, if needed, with cinnamon, fresh black pepper, herbs or spices.
6. Inspect the preheated oven, then stir halfway through all the cooking procedures for the period (see above recommended times).
7. Roast until your ideal level of crispiness and caramelization is achieved. Pierce the sensitivity with a fork or a knife.
8. Serve instantly.

## 10.7. Christmas Magic Bars

Preparation Time: 4 hours 15 min | Servings: 3 | Difficulty: Medium

**Ingredients**

- Pork belly, 1.2 kg
- Shaoxing wine, 1/2 tbsp, optional
- To taste, rock salt.

Seasonings:

- Salt, 3½ tsp
- Sugar, 2 tsp
- Five-spice powder, 1/2 tsp

**Directions**

1. For seasonings: mix the salt with both the sugar and other five-spice powder well. Set it back.

2. Use a knife for scraping-out some impurities and fur. Now rinse thoroughly. Blanch the ingredients in boiling water for around 15 minutes, before 60 to 70% is finished, or till the skin becomes softened. Drain them well and clean with paper towels. Using the needles, give the rind, holes as many as you can. Turn around to the other side and cut into a few meat slices to better absorb all the seasonings.

3. Brush wine on bacon. Let it rest for a moment. Coat the beef equally with the seasonings. Making sure there are no seasonings left on the rind, or the five-spice powder will make it darken.

4. Wrap the bacon with foil and keep the rind unwrapped. Put in the refrigerator, let the air dry in the oven overnight.

5. Preheat the oven to 200C or 395F.

6. Remove the pork from the refrigerator and remove the foil. Let it rest at room temperature

for some time. Poke the rind uniformly with the needles again. Clean wiping. Season this same rind with some rock salt. Bake into the preheated oven for around 30 minutes (note: convection oven is used in my case. If the oven is normal, then bake it for 45 minutes.) Raise the temp. To 220C/430F, bake again for 10-15 minutes or till you have enough crackling. Note Grill the rind till it is uniformly blistered and browned.)

## 10.8 Grilled veg sandwiches in the oven

Preparation Time: 14 min | Servings: 4 | Difficulty: Easy

**Ingredients**

For filling

- Onion chopped, 1/4 cup
- Tomato chopped, 1/4 cup
- Bell peppers or Capsicum, chopped, 1/4 cup
- Carrot grated, 1/4 cup
- Salt as required
- Cumin powder roasted, 1 tsp
- Black pepper powder, 1/2 tsp
- Chaat masala, 1/2 tsp
- Tomato sauce/ketchup, 1 or 2 tsp

For sandwich

- Bread slices, 8
- Butter, 4 tsp
- Green chutney, 4 tsp
- Tomato sauce/ketchup, 4 tsp
- Vegetable filling, 3 to 4 tsp (for each sandwich)

- Cheese slices, 4
- Onion / Tomato slices, 8
- Black pepper powder (to sprinkle) and some chaat masala &

**Directions**

Sandwich filling.

1. Add and mix the vegetables in a bowl.
2. Insert cumin with black pepper, some chaat masala and the tomato sauce with some salt.
3. Mix all the items.
4. Take two slices of bread, then apply butter on one side of the slices of bread. Spread some ketchup on one slice of bread while on the other side, use some green chutney.
5. Then spread the lining of the sandwich.
6. Place a piece of cheese on top, then sprinkle some chat masala and black pepper in powder form.
7. Place two slices of tomato or onion on top.
8. Cover the buttered side of the sandwich on top.
9. Place them onto the grill rack and then cook for 2 minutes (in grill mode).
10. Flip them back and barbecue for another two minutes after 2 minutes.
11. Crunchy sandwiches of grilled veg are waiting to be served.

## 10.9 Oven-Roasted Spicy Fries

Preparation Time: 50 min | Servings: 4-6 | Difficulty: Easy

**Ingredients**

- Vegetable oil spray to make the pan nonstick as needed
- Unpeeled russet potatoes, 2 pounds wedges.

- Canola oil, 2 tbsps
- Red chili powder as desired

**Directions**

1. Preheat the oven to a temperature of 450 ° F.
2. Spray with some kind of nonstick spray on a wide-rimmed baking sheet.
3. In a wide tub, toss the potato wedges along with canola oil.
4. Sprinkle the potato wedges evenly with salt and black pepper; scatter over the lined baking sheet in one layer.
5. Roast the potato wedges till soft and brown in patches, regularly rotating for around 45 minutes.
6. Finally, sprinkle some salt and pepper, then serve hot.

## 10.10 Garlic roasted potatoes

Preparation Time: 40 min | Servings: 5-6 | Difficulty: Easy

**Ingredients**

- Diced potatoes, 4 cups 1/2-inch cubes
- Olive oil, 2 tbsp
- Kosher salt, 1 tsp
- Paprika 1 tsp
- Garlic powder, 1/2 tsp
- Coarsely ground black pepper, 1/2 tsp
- Onion powder, ¼ tsp

### Directions

1. Preheat your oven to 425 ° F.
2. Toss the diced potatoes with some oil, cinnamon, paprika and garlic powder, along with some pepper and onion powder before all the potatoes have been sufficiently covered with spices.
3. Spread in a single layer over the baking sheet. Roast them for 20 minutes, stir and proceed to roast again for 15 minutes or till crispy from the outside and soft from the inside (the baking period can differ significantly based on how big or small you slice the potatoes).
4. Enjoy.

## 10.11 Roasted butternut squash

Preparation Time: 45 min | Servings: 2 | Difficulty: Easy

### Ingredients

- Butternut squash, 1 large
- Olive oil, 1 tbsp
- Pinch of salt
- Freshly ground black pepper as per your taste.

### Directions

1. Preheat the oven up to 425 F when using a convection oven and 450 F when using a conventional oven.
2. Check the pot's directions to peel and extract the seeds of butternut squash and make 1-inch cubes.
3. Place cubes inside a medium or a wide mixing bowl and add no more than 1 tbsp. Of olive oil to cover it properly, sprinkle some salt and black pepper or other some kind of other seasonings and spices, if needed. Cut cubed squash in one layer on a half-leaf pan should be lined with parchment/silicone baking sheet (in case you have smaller, let say 13×9-inch

sheet pans, then you would need 2 pans). If you don't get interested in using oil, a silicone baking pad is particularly useful to avoid sticking.

4. Roast uncovered for around 15 minutes, rotate the cubes, transfer to the oven, then again cook until the fork is penetrated with no resistance, around 15 to 20 further minutes will be required.

5.

## 10.12 Oven Roasted Cauliflower Recipe

Preparation Time: 55 min | Servings: 6 | Difficulty: Easy

**Ingredients**

- Cauliflower large, 1
- Olive oil, 2 tbsps
- Paprika, 1 tsp
- Salt, 1/4 tsp
- Minced garlic cloves, 3
- Parsley flakes, 2 tbsps

**Directions**

1. Preheat the oven to 450 ° F
2. Split the cauliflower into big pieces and put them inside a large cup. Combine the oil, paprika with some salt in a small bowl; sprinkle over the cauliflower.
3. Mix well and spray the cauliflower as uniformly as possible.
4. In a separate dish, mix the sliced garlic with some parsley flakes and put aside. Spread the cauliflower over a 10 x 15 x 1 sized baking sheet and put inside the preheated oven, uncovered.
5. Bake for around 10 minutes, then extract from the oven, then add the garlic with parsley flakes in it; mix well the cauliflower to combine everything evenly.

6. Put in the oven for another 10-15 minutes or till the cauliflower becomes crispy and gently browned. Stir over during the cooking once or twice.

7. When the cauliflower is cooked, extract from the oven. Now serve it hot.

## 10.13 Brussel sprout parmesan

### Ingredients

- Raw brussels sprouts, one lb washed and ends trimmed
- Extra virgin olive oil, 2 tbsp
- Freshly shredded parmesan cheese, heaping cup 1/4
- Breadcrumbs plain panko, 1/4 cup
- Granulated garlic, 1 tsp (powdered garlic is fine as well)
- Sea salt, 1/2 tsp
- Ground black pepper, 1/4 tsp

### Directions

1. For traditional oven toasting: Preheat your oven to 450 For at 425 F in case of convection oven) Add the halved Brussels sprouts (washed) into a 9 x 13 sized glass or maybe a corning-ware baking dish; now add some oil and stir to get a smooth coat. Don't overfill the dish. You need one layer of Brussels sprouts. In case you wish to double the recipe, use the 2nd baking dish to prevent overcrowding.

2. In a shallow cup, mix the remaining ingredients: including parmesan, breadcrumbs, and garlic pieces, salt and pepper.

3. Add the mixture of parmesan to the sprouts, then stir.

4. Roast Brussels sprouts for about 20 minutes, stirring in the center. This will bring your Brussels in fried condition and make it brown & crispy from the outside, but always use a little green.

## 10.14 Spaghetti squash

Preparation Time: 50 min | Servings: 4 | Difficulty: Easy

### Ingredients

- Spaghetti squash 1 (2-3 pounds)
- Olive oil, 2 tbsps
- Kosher salt with some freshly ground black pepper, as per taste.

### Directions

1. Preheat the oven to 375 ° F. Slightly oil the baking sheet or use a nonstick spray coat.
2. Break the squash into half, start from the stem and end to the tail, then remove the seeds. Drizzle some olive oil and then season with some salt and pepper according to the taste.
3. Place the squash such that the cut side is down on the already prepared baking dish. Put in the oven and toast until tender, around 35-45 minutes, is required.
4. Remove from the oven and let it rest until it is cold enough to treat.
5. Scrape the flesh with a fork to produce long threads.

## 10.15 Asian-Inspired Shepherd's Pie

Preparation Time: 45 min | Servings: 8 | Difficulty: Medium

### Ingredients

- Diced carrots, 1/2 cup
- Diced celery, 1/2 cup
- Diced onion, 1/2 cup
- Diced green onion, 1/2 cup
- Minced garlic cloves, 4
- Shiitake mushrooms 1 cup, sliced in half
- Shelled edamame, 1 cup

- Dry white wine, 1/2 cup
- Leftover turkey meat, 1 pound, pulled apart or chopped off the bone.
- Gravy, 4 cups
- Soy sauce, 1/8 cup
- Sesame oil, 1 tbsp
- Mashed potatoes, 6 cups
- Olive oil, 2 tbsps
- Toasted sesame seeds or crumbled nori seeds for garnish.
- Salt and pepper, as per taste

**Directions**

1. Preheat your oven to a temperature of 450 ° F.
2. Sautee the vegetables gently in a medium pot. When soft, add the wine, then cook before the scent of alcohol wears away. Place the turkey meat, then add the gravel, soy sauce and some sesame oil; it will make a Nice seasoning flavor for the blend.
3. Spread the filling inside a 12-by-8-inch saucepan. Spread the mashed potatoes, use a spatula to get it uniform on top. If you want to maximize the tightness, drag a fork over the top to build further grooves. If you prefer, blot with sugar.
4. Bake for approximately thirty minutes. Switch the fan on in case you have a convection type oven. You can use the broiler choice to render a decent crust if the top isn't so brown as you like after 30 minutes. But track it to make sure it doesn't burn.
5. When you have a perfect look, encourage the casserole to settle down for around 15 minutes before serving.

# Chapter 11: Bread recipe

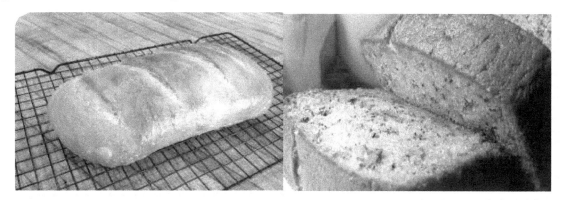

## 11.1 Homemade Bread

Preparation Time: 2 hrs. 30 min | Servings: 3 | Difficulty: Easy

**Ingredients**

- Warm water, 1 quart
- Sugar, ⅓ cup
- Yeast, 1 ybsp
- Salt, 1 tbsp
- Vegetable oil, ½ cup
- Flour, 3 cups to start, then sufficient for making the dough not gluey.

**Directions**

1. Take warm water and dissolve the yeast and sugar in it. It depends on your choice to do this in one cup and then add the remaining warm water into the batch.
2. Add iodine, vegetable oil and about 3 cups of flour with the yeast mixture.
3. Insert more flour, half to one cup at a time, till the dough is no longer stuck to the surface of the tub.
4. Place the dough on the counter and then knead until it is soft and elastic.

5. Put in a greased dish, rotating once to cover the whole dough mixture.

6. Let the dough rise till it is double, now hit it down.

7. Let the dough grow again, then strike it again.

8. Grease the bread pans and mound the dough into the loaves.

9. Place the melted margarine, or you can also use vegetable oil over the top of the loaves.

10. Prick each loaf from several places.

11. Allow rising to make it double.

12. Bake at 350 °F for 30 minutes or till packed. Enjoy.

## 11.2 Cinnamon flavored banana bread

Preparation Time: 70 min | Servings: 7-8 | Difficulty: Medium

**Ingredients**

- All-purpose flour, 2 cups, spoon & smoothed
- Baking soda, 1 tsp
- Salt, 1/4 tsp
- Cinnamon, 1/2 tsp, ground
- Unsalted butter, 1/2 cup, softened at room temperature.
- Brown sugar, 3/4 cup, Light or dark
- Eggs, 2 large, at room temperature
- Plain yogurt, 1/3 cup
- Bananas, 2 cups, mashed
- Pure vanilla extract, 1 tsp

- Pecans or walnuts, 3/4 cup, sliced.

**Directions**

1. Shift the oven rack in such a way that it is at the bottom third place. Now preheat the oven to about 350º F (177 º C). Grease the loaf pan of about nine into 5-inch, or you can also use a nonstick spray for coating. Set it aside.

2. In a big cup, mix rice, baking soda, some salt and cinnamon. Using a portable or stand blender with either a paddle or whisk attachment, blend the butter and brown sugar fast till it is soft and fluffy for around 2 minutes. At a moderate pace, mix the eggs one by one, beating quickly after each insertion. Mix in yogurt, the mashed bananas and the vanilla extract at a medium pace until mixed. Steadily beat the remaining dry ingredients and wet ingredients using the blender, working at low speed till the flour pockets exist. Don't over mix it. Fold the seeds if you need them.

3. Place the batter in the already prepared baking pan, then bake for about 60-65 mins. Cover the bread loosely with aluminum foil after 30 mins. To prevent from being too brown from the top and the sides. A toothpick stranded in the middle of the loaf would come out clear when your bread is ready. Take out the bread from the oven, then cool fully inside the pan place on the wire rack.

4. Cover and keep the banana bread for storage at room temperature for about two days, or you can keep it up to 1 week in the refrigerator. Banana bread tastes much better on day two once the spices have been mixed.

## 11.3 Brown bread

Preparation Time: 44 min | Servings:2-3 | Difficulty: Medium

**Ingredients**

- All-purpose flour, 2.25 cups
- Whole wheat flour, ¾ cup
- Water, 1 cup

- Dry active yeast, ½ tbsp
- Sunflower oil, 2 tbsps, organic cold-pressed
- Regular sugar, 1 tbsp
- Rock salt, 1 tsp

**Directions**

Proofing Yeast

1. Heat about 1 cup of water.
2. Add one Tbsp of sugar and then dry active yeast.
3. Swirl and then activate the yeast.
4. It normally requires about 10 minutes.
5. Kneading Dough of Brown Bread in a Container
6. Sift both flours with some salt in a huge, wide bowl, or you can use a big rim/plate.
7. Add now the proofed yeast with oil.
8. Mix all the products.
9. Then start kneading the dough.
10. When the dough is soft, add more starch.
11. When it feels dusty, add some water.
12. Keep kneading until you have a smooth dough that does not break when extended.

Kneading Dough of Brown Bread with a stand mixer

1. Apply the flour and some salt to the dish.
2. Mix flour and the salt for a few seconds at speed 1.
3. Add the mixture of yeast and the oil, then knead the dough at speed 2.
4. Keep kneading for about 2 minutes and look for the dough.
5. Add some lukewarm water if the dough seems dry.

6. Add some flour in case the dough is wet.

7. Continue kneading for another 2-3 minutes at speed two until you have a nice and foldable dough.

Leavening Dough of Brown Bread

1. Rub oil or some water all over the ready dough and then leave for about 2-3 hours in a wrapped bowl.

2. Remove the dough, then punch it after 2-3 hours, now deflate it gently.

3. Roll out a single small log of the dough.

4. Take the corners off on all sides of the rolled bread loaf.

5. Put the bread now in a 9x5 inches oiled loaf pan, having tucked sides facing downwards.

6. Wrap the loaf pan, leave this dough for about 40 minutes, or be for 1 hour.

7. Preheat the oven to 180 ° Celsius or 350 ° F.

8. Bake the loaf now for about 35-40 minutes or bake it till the bread sounds hollow.

9. Put the bread on either a rack or plate.

10. Serve your brown bread either warm or refrigerated.

## 11.4 Simple banana bread

### Ingredients

- All-purpose flour 2 cups, spoon & smoothed
- Baking soda 1 tsp
- Salt 1/4 tsp
- Cinnamon 1/2 tsp, ground
- Unsalted butter 1/2 cup, softened at room temperature
- Brown sugar 3/4 cup, Light or dark

- Eggs 2 large, at room temperature
- Plain yogurt 1/3 cup
- Bananas 2 cups, mashed
- Pure vanilla extract one tsp
- Pecans or walnuts 3/4 cup, sliced and it's optional

**Instructions**

1. Shift the oven rack in such a way that it is at the bottom third place. Now preheat the oven to about 350º F (177 º C). Grease the loaf pan of about nine into 5-inch, or you can also use a nonstick spray for coating. Set it aside.

2. In a big bowl, mix together rice, baking soda, some salt and cinnamon. By using a portable or stand blender with either a paddle or may be whisk attachment, blend the butter and the brown sugar together at fast speed till it is soft and fluffy for around 2 minutes. At a moderate pace, mix the eggs one by one, beating quickly after each insertion. Mix in yogurt, the mashed bananas and in the vanilla extract at a medium pace until mixed. Steadily beat the remaining dry ingredients along with wet ingredients using the blender, working at low speed till the flour pockets exist. Don't over mix it. Fold the seeds if you need them.

3. Place the batter in the already prepared baking pan, then bake for about 60-65 mins. Cover the bread loosely with aluminum foil after 30 mins. To prevent from being too brown from the top and the sides. A toothpick stranded in the middle of the loaf would come out clear when your bread is ready. Take out the bread from the oven, then allow it to cool fully inside the pan place on the wire rack.

4. Cover and keep the banana bread for storage at the room temperature for about two days, or you can keep it up to 1 week in the refrigerator. Banana bread tastes much better on day two once the spices have been mixed together.

# Chapter 12: Miscellaneous

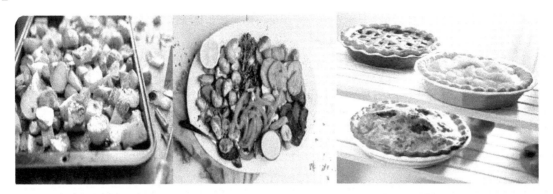

## 12.1 Oven-roasted root veggies

Preparation Time: 25 min | Servings: 6 | Difficulty: Easy

**Ingredients:**

- Baking apples, 5 ½ cups, sliced
- Lemon juice, 1 ½ tbsp, fresh
- Lemon zest, ¼ tsp, grated
- Sugar, ¼ cup, granulated
- Cinnamon, ½ tsp, ground
- Salt, ¼ tsp
- Rolled oats, ½ cup
- Packed brown sugar, 2/3 cup
- Flour, 1/3 cup
- Baking powder, ¼ tsp
- Margarine, ½ cup, you can also use butter

**Directions**

1. Preheat the oven to about 350 °F with a convection environment, 375 °F with a traditional oven.

2. Place the apples in a big bowl, then sprinkle with the lemon juice and the zest. Mix sugar, salt and then cinnamon together in a small bowl. Spray over apples. Stir gently to moisten the sugar mixture and put the apples in an 11/7- or 9/9-inch baking tray.

3. Mix oats, brown sugar, flour and the baking powder together in a medium dish. Add margarine and then work using two forks or even a pastry cutter to produce a crumbly paste. Sprinkle the apples uniformly in the jar.

4. Toast inside the preheated convection oven for 40 minutes and 45 minutes in case of a conventional oven or until the surface is bubbling and finely browned.

5. Serve hot, or you can also serve cold using ice cream or even whipped cream if needed.

## 12.2 Stacked Enchilada Pie

Preparation Time: 80 min | Servings: 8 | Difficulty: Medium

**Ingredients**

- Onion 1, skinned and chopped.
- Red bell peppers 2, washed, stemmed, seeded, and sliced.
- Garlic 2 cloves, skinned and pressed
- Cumin seeds, 2 tbsp
- Salad oil 1 tsp
- Corn kernels one package, frozen and thawed.
- Black beans two cans washed and drained.
- Fresh cilantro 1/2 cup, chopped.
- Red chili, 1 can sauce.

- Flour tortillas, 8
- Pepper jack 3 cups, shredded
- cotija/feta cheese, 1 1/2 cups, smashed
- Avocado 1, firm-ripe
- Cilantro sprigs, Fresh and rinsed.

**Directions**

1. In the nonstick pan of approx. 5 to 6 quart using high flame, regularly mix the onion, the bell peppers, garlic and then cumin seeds in 1 tsp of oil till the onion is loose for 5-7 minutes. Stir in maize, beans, and then chopped cilantro; now remove the pan from heat.

2. Put the chili sauce into a rimmed pizza pan or 12-inch, or you can also use a pie pan of 10-inch. Dip the tortilla in the sauce to coat all sides lightly; cut the tortilla, and let the excess sauce drain back into the plate. Put tortilla inside an oiled cheesecake tray of 10-inch having a removable rim of about 3 inches. Spread vegetable filling (almost 1 cup) on the tortilla. Sprinkle uniformly with jack cheese of about 1/3 cup and then three tbsp of cotija cheese. Repeat the layers, creating a total of 7, top with the last tortilla. Reserve the leftover chili sauce and the remaining jack and then cotija cheese. Cover the plate with the oiled sheet of foil on the oiled side off. Put the pan inside a rimmed 10-15-inch baking pan.

3. Bake in 350° F standard, or you can also use a 325° F convection oven for about 30 minutes. Remove the lid and continue cooking until it's hot (160°) in the middle, 30-40 minutes longer.

4. Before eating, in a microwave-safe bowl, put it inside a microwave, oven having full-power or having 100% heat, now heat the remaining chili sauce for almost about 20 to 30 secs. Pit, peel, and chop the avocado.

5. Take a knife and run it between the pie and the pan to loosen. Uncover the rim, put the pie on the plate and drizzle with the chili sauce. Arrange the avocado slices in the pie loop, scatter with the remaining jack and the cotija cheeses and then garnish with the cilantro sprigs. Break the wedges to serve.

## 12.3 Golden rice crisps

Preparation Time: 20 min | Servings: 4 | Difficulty: Easy

**Ingredient**

- Rice flour, ½ cup
- Cornstarch, ¼ cup
- Turmeric ½ tsp, grounded and dried.
- Coconut milk, ¼ cup, canned
- Green onion, 2 tbsps, thinly chopped, including tops
- Salad oil, 1 tbsp
- Seasoned fish sauce

**Directions**

1. Mix the rice flour, cornstarch and turmeric inside a dish. Add 1 cup of water with the coconut milk, then whisk to mix. Stir the green onion.
2. Place a nonstick pan of about 12-inch (10 inches across the bottom) over a high flame. When the pan is heated, add one Tsp of oil and move to the pan's bottom.
3. Stir in the rice flour mixture to blend. Place 1/2 cup of the batter in the pan at once while turning the pan to fill the whole bottom equally.
4. Cook till the crêpe becomes browned and crispy on the bottom, for about 3-5 minutes. Switch to a 14/17 inches baking sheet with a flat spatula. Repeat it for two more crêpes and add to the sheet with a single layer when cooked.
5. Bake it in a 350° F standard or convection oven till the crêpes are fluffy, for 8–12 minutes. Transfer to the racks to cool off.
6. Break the bits and dunk in prepared fish sauce to consume.

## 12.4 Apple and Endive Salad with Honey Vinaigrette

Preparation Time: 5 min | Servings: 1 | Difficulty: Easy

**Ingredient**

1. Orange blossom 2 tbsps, you can use other mild honey.
2. Champagne vinegar 2 tbsps, or it can be white wine vinegar.
3. Grape-seed oil 1 tbsp
4. Red or white Belgian endive 2 heads, washed, ends trimmed.
5. Sweet apple 1, washed, cored, and thinly chopped lengthwise.
6. Pecan halves ⅓ cup, grilled and coarsely sliced.
7. Blue cheese 2 ounces, smashed.
8. Salt as required

**Directions**

1. Mix honey and the vinegar with oil inside a large bowl.
2. Now add the endive, apple, pecans and the blue cheese, then blend softly to coat.
3. Add salt according to taste, Enjoy!

## 12.5 Endive casserole

Preparation Time: 1 day, 1 hour, 20 min | Servings: 4-6 | Difficulty: Difficult

**Ingredients**

- Fennel with stalks six heads
- Belgian endive, 3 heads
- Butter, ¼ cup, olive oil can also be used
- Prosciutto, 3 ounces, thinly chopped
- all-purpose flour, 3 tbsps

- Chicken broth, 2 cups, fat-skimmed chicken
- Whipping cream, 1 cup
- Gorgonzola, 8 ounces, smashed

**Directions**

1. Cut off soft green fennel leaves; clean, drain, cover in a towel, put inside a plastic bag, and then chill for about one day.

2. Remove and dispose of stalks, the root ends, as well as any damaged part from fennel heads. Rinse the heads and split halfway through the widest dimension. Remove and discard the root ends, which are discolored and any kind of leaves discolored from the endive. Break the heads into two halves lengthwise.

3. Melt two tbsp of butter in a pan of about 10-12-inch over medium-high flame. Lay quite enough fennel that suits, cut horizontally, in the pan, then brown slightly, for about 3-4 minutes; rotate and brown the curved sides, for 3-4 minutes longer. If the butter continues to scorch, apply 1 to 2 tbsp of water at once. As browned, move the fennel, sliced sideways, a shallow casserole of 3-quart or 9/13-inch baking dish, and the remaining brown bits.

4. When all the fennel is browned, put the endive, cut side down, in the frying pan and then brown for 3 to 4 minutes, then add 1–2 tbsps of water if it starts to scorch. Switch over and brown at the tip, 3 or 4 minutes longer.

5. Remove the pan from the heat and pass the endives to the cutting board. Break the halves in half lengthwise. Tea prosciutto cuts into broad, thin strips. Wrap the endive pieces with the same prosciutto. Fit the endive pieces equally between the fennel pieces in the casserole.

6. In the unclean pan over a high flame, dissolve the remaining 2 tbsp. Melted butter, then add flour and mix until lightly browned, around 2 minutes. Remove from heat, then mix in the broth and milk. Transfer pan to high flame and whisk before boiling; simmer and mix for 2 minutes. Attach 1/3 cup of cheese and whisk till it is molten. Pour the sauce uniformly over the fennel and the endive, covering both surfaces. Cover firmly with tape.

7. Bake inside a 375 ° standard or convection oven for around 40 minutes, till the fennel is soft when penetrated.

8. Uncover the remaining cheese and then bake for about 20 minutes till browned. Chop the reserved fennel leaves for 1/2 cup and scatter over the casserole. Serve yourself hot and enjoy it.

# Conclusion

This cookbook provided you detailed information about the usage of a convection oven. You may now know why convection oven is nowadays very famous for cooking purposes. There is fan and exhaust mechanism in the convection oven that a conventional oven does not provide. You must have learned how it is different and better from conventional oven cooking. Convection ovens look the same in all styles and can be gas or electric. The contrast between them is that traditional oven heat is stationary and grows from the oven's bottom. Fans from a convection oven blow the fire, so the air distributes all over the oven's interior.

The book also provided many recipes, including delicious and easy to make recipes of chicken, turkey, fish, bread, pizza, beef and lamb etc. Now you must have learned how to work with a convection oven, when to use it and when not to use it. Stay motivated and keep on making delicious c recipes in the convection oven. Because after reading this book, nothing can stop you from becoming perfect at cooking and baking in convection oven.

Lightning Source UK Ltd.
Milton Keynes UK
UKHW032224211220
375683UK00007B/742